Better
WITH
a Bag than
IN
a Bag

From the Brink of Death to Recovery through
Humour & Inspiration

by
Jo-Ann L. Tremblay

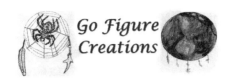

Ottawa Canada
Go Figure Creations
www.potentialsmanagement.com
Blog: joannltremblay.wordpress.com
facebook: Jo-Ann L. Tremblay
Twitter: @joanntremblay

1st Edition

First Go Figure Creations electronic edition November 24, 2012

Amazon.com edition November 26, 2012

Designed by Go Figure Creations

Cover design copyright © 2012 Go Figure Creations

Cover painting copyright © 2012 Jo-Ann L. Tremblay

Author's Photo by Joan Anderson

ISBN-13: 978-0-9809009-1-0

DEDICATION

This is for you Mark. Thanks for everything and all the beyond's you've been and done for Percy & Me.

To Richard for all that you are, and being there for Mark, Percy and Me.

Thanks to the children, their life partners and the grandchildren of my blended family, for sharing the music of your hearts.

Finally, I dedicate this book to you all, thanks for allowing Percy and Me to be part of your lives.

Table of Contents

Table of Contents

Table of Contents

Table of Contents

Prologue

As adventures go, Jo-Ann L. Tremblay has had many. But, nothing prepared her for the odyssey she embarked on in 2008.

This is the real-life story of an ordinary woman taking a stand against an extraordinary nemesis called diverticular disease. The story follows her as she navigates through a myriad of doctors, diagnostic tests and procedures, only to find herself lost in the mysterious landscape of misdiagnosis.

Who will help her . . .

What does she do to save her life . . .

Time is running out!

PART 1

Things Are Going Downhill

It is the Master of Self who is the masterpiece; the life lived is the canvas that reveals the Master's great works. — Jo-Ann L. Tremblay

Better with a bag than in a bag. — Mark Henderson

Coming Out of the Water Closet

The night it happened, Mark, my husband, was downtown on Elgin Street in Ottawa Canada at Maxwell's Bistro & Club, rocking to the music of Johnny Vegas and his All-Star band. Beki, second-oldest daughter of our blended family, sings female vocal, and we enjoy the performances. I was feeling physically terrible, an ongoing way of life it seemed by then, and I couldn't make it out that evening. I sure would have loved to have been there making enough noise "to wake the dead". (This thought would come back to haunt in the hours that followed.) My life seemed out of control, I needed to be close to a toilet at all times. I was in pain. I was tired. My body and my life simply seemed to be telling me how much things had changed. Sitting here at my computer now, last summer feels like another world away. It's the right time to start getting it all out of my brain and onto paper where it can be more understood, explained, and edited. It's time to get my story out of my body in the hopes that I don't have to carry the weight of it around for the rest of my days, to make sense of it before I fully step out into my new life, my new normal.

Truth be told, making sense of it bothers me so. Can one actually make sense of the senseless? Certain things happen because of bad genes and bad luck — plain and simple. Wrong confidences, wrong diagnoses, misplaced trusts: shit happens. You can't explain it because, from time to time, bad things happen just because they do. During the course of a lifetime, yes, shit happens and weird stuff does too.

"It all happens for a reason." "There's more for you to do." "You're not meant to go yet." That's what they say. Makes me laugh, makes me cry, makes me angry and mostly it makes me think. At times, a part of me wants to forget all of this. I've got bad stuff in my mind. But there's another part of me that wants to put it out there and let the light shine on it. Every part of it is jaw-dropping amazing, horrible, incredible, and it blows my mind every time I think about it.

It's time to lay it all out, come out of the water closet so to speak, as I get through it bit by bit, jotting it down in the hopes that it will eventually be my purgation of emotions, my purification that will bring about spiritual renewal. At the very least, my release from tension.

So here goes!

Do not dwell on what you believe you are doing wrong; instead, focus on what you know you are doing right and you will take flight. — Jo-Ann L. Tremblay

The Long Hard Journey

It's hard to pinpoint the actual beginning of my intestinal problems. As far back as I can remember I've had issues. In fact, most of my family has had to deal with the poop on poops for four generations now, that we're aware of. We sure have some great genes, but, we sure do have some nasty ones, too. My grandmother, my father, my mother, my sister, and my son have all fought the good fight. Intestinal issues range from IBS (Irritable Bowel Syndrome), colitis, Crohn's disease, leaky gut, celiac disease, and my personal contributions: ulcerated colitis and diverticular disease. It's interesting sitting around the dinner table when we're altogether. We are the First Family of Poopology, we are the amazing bombastic flatulent high flyers. Creating the menu is a real feat of culinary management, every single bowel in the room must be considered and catered to. Oh, the joy of cooking!

It's time to take a few steps back and take another look at what led up to the life-altering event that almost sealed my fate. I have my illness story — my individualized version. What I have discovered after meeting with many people is that each has her own unique and horrifying version of suffering, journeys that are filled with all the pain and humiliation of what a bowel disease can do to a person and the quality of her life.

Although I have always had a delicate bowel system, my downhill path to disaster started in 2008. With each passing month, the pain in my abdomen was becoming more debilitating. As time passed beyond the pain, there were, of course, my frequent bowel movements. Well . . . let's just say I knew where every toilet was in every facility, everywhere.

What should I eat, what should I not eat? "Thanks for the dinner invitation. Yes, I can eat vegetables but not tomatoes with seeds in it. No, I can't eat green, red or yellow peppers. I'd better stay away from spices. No, I shouldn't have any coarse pepper. Oh, there's nuts in that. Well, it looks delicious but I think I'll pass. Oh, by the way, could you tell me where your toilet facilities are? Thanks."

And that's was just the beginning. After picking so many wonderful things out of my food and placing them on the side of the plate, it would be just the time for me to start eating what remained of what I thought my system could digest and then . . . "Oh, excuse me. I'll be back in a moment. The bathroom is just down the hall you say? Yes? Thank you."

My world was becoming smaller and smaller. There were the invitations to visit family, friends, or to enjoy a day with the children and grandchildren. "Thanks for the invitation, but I'm so tired, I think I'll have to pass. Have a nice time though." "Geez, it's early, but I'm just so exhausted I think we have to leave now." "Why don't you go out and enjoy yourself, I'll just stay in bed and rest awhile." Thank goodness we have an en suite bathroom.

"It's hot isn't it? Don't you find it a bit warm? Oh, you're right. I do have a fever. It's pretty low grade, though. Gosh, it's awfully warm. Oh my goodness, it's really cold isn't it? Are you cold? I think we need to turn up the thermostat. Oh, it's not that cold? Oh, you're right. I do have a fever. It's low grade, though. Well, it's been a couple of months now that I've had this fever. Be back in a minute. Just have to go to the washroom. Again."

There's pain in my butt and everywhere else in my body. "I sure would love to sit on the floor with you, honey, and play with your trucks, but Gramma Jo just can't get down there. If I do, I don't think I can get back up. I think I'll sit on this soft couch. Gramma Jo has a sore body today. I just can't bend over honey. Could you pick that up for me? Thanks. Oh, that's just too high. Could you reach that for me, please? Go see Dramps. Gramma Jo just has to go to the potty. See you in a few minutes."

***

"Yes, Doctor, I feel just awful. I'm going to the bathroom to eliminate, well . . . It's about ten times a day now on average. But there are some days when it's more than this."

"Well, Jo-Ann your colonoscopy shows that you have quite severe diverticular disease. We're going to put you on an anti-inflammatory prescription. And as for the low-grade fever, your blood tests are showing a high white cell count. This happens when a person is fighting an infection or dealing with pain. I'll also prescribe an antibiotic. Take seven anti-inflammatory pills per day, and make sure you complete the whole antibiotic prescription."

***

"Doctor, it's been six weeks. The abdominal pain is getting worse. I'm running to the bathroom more than ten times a day now. The low-grade fever disappeared for a couple of days, then came back, and I'm still feverish."

"Continue to take your anti-inflammatory medication, but I want you to increase them to nine pills a day. Your colonoscopy also indicated that you have ulcerated colitis. Once we get the intestinal infection calmed down, your bowels will calm down. I think we'd better prescribe more antibiotics."

***

"Hello Doctor, it's now been six more weeks since I was in your office. Well, I'm now going to the bathroom so many times during the course of a day, I don't bother counting anymore. I still have the low-grade fever. I am unable to regulate my body temperature. Sometimes I'm really warm, and other times I'm really cold. My body pain is quite intense. Even my hair hurts some mornings. Have you ever heard of someone's hair hurting? I'm so tired. And the chronic pain has completely affected my quality of life. I really feel I'm surviving, but I'm sure not thriving. I think I'd like to be referred to a gastroenterologist. Something really bad is happening in there. I need help."

"Up your anti-inflammatory medication, Jo-Ann. I think we'll try another antibiotic. Here's your prescription."

"But Doctor, I'm not getting any better. Don't you think I should see a gastroenterologist?"

You're Weird & God Hates You

November 2010 and all is not well. While sitting at my computer that Wednesday, all heck started breaking loose in my body. *Oh my, I'm so cold, I'm shivering. I can't even type anymore. What's wrong with me? My thoughts were running in every direction at this point. Oh, I'm so sick. Something is definitely wrong with me. My thoughts are now turning to slight panic as I picked up the phone. No one's answering at the doctor's office. I think I need to go to the Urgent Care Clinic.*

I was lying on the examination table when the Urgent Care Doctor walked in with a file in his hand. He took one glance at me, and a look of concern clouded his face.

"You're not here for a hang nail. I'm going to examine you. Oh, you're tender here. Oh. Sorry. Everywhere in the abdomen. You're quite distended. Go next door. I'm ordering up blood and urine tests. I think we have a real issue here. Then, go home and wait by the phone. I'll call you with the results and my recommendations."

I sat waiting by the phone in a state of hot and cold, with lightning bolts of jagged pain igniting every nerve and cell throughout my body. Sure enough, an hour later the phone rings.

"Ms. Tremblay, your white cell count is very high, and the blood and urine results are quite concerning. Swing around to Urgent Care, pick up your results — or have someone do this for you — then go straight to the hospital. Right away!"

"Wow! What an awful looking hospital room. It looks like a room that's designed to be hosed down, Mom," said my son Richard when he arrived in my temporary room. "You're not looking very good. You're still so cold. Can I get you another blanket? Is there anything we can do for you?"

"Nope. I think I'll just lie quiet for a while. They'll be taking me down soon for a CT Scan. They've taken a lot of blood and urine. We'll just have to wait for the results. They told me they're moving me to a permanent room on another floor soon."

For a week, while hooked up to oxygen, I had an intravenous line containing four types of powerful antibiotics that dripped into my veins constantly. I underwent many tests, my white cell count was not good at all. Unfortunately, even with a great medical team and state-of-the-art medical technology such as CT Scan and ultrasound, the team of doctors at the hospital were unable to pinpoint what my health issue was.

During the course of my seven-day hospital ordeal, the doctor on my case stated, "It's a mystery disease. We cannot find the source of the problem. You're weird and God hates you."

"Sheesh, thanks Doc. Weird I can agree with, but really, I don't think God hates me."

After a week of morphine for the pain, and loaded up with antibiotics, I was sent home with no definitive diagnosis. I apparently had been suffering with sepsis, systemic inflammatory response syndrome (SIRS). All the symptoms and test results pointed in that direction, but apparently, no one knew why. In retrospect, this inability to diagnose the source of the problem is still mind-blowing to me to this day.

While attending the follow up doctor's visit with my general practitioner after the hospital discharge, I asked questions. "Okay Doc, what is septicaemia, and how could I have gotten it?"

"Well Jo-Ann, it is basically blood poisoning. It is a bacteria in the blood that often occurs with severe infections. There is no doubt that it's a serious, life-threatening infection that can get worse very quickly. It can arise from infections throughout the body, including infections in the lungs, abdomen, and urinary tract. It may come before or at the same time as infections of the bone, central nervous system, heart and other tissues."

"So how would I have gotten to this point?" I asked.

"Well, you can get a blood infection from an open and unattended wound."

"A wound. What kind of wound?"

"Oh, an open wound on the battlefield that is weeping and left unattended, for example."

"Really. Well I don't even have a scratch, so we can eliminate that source."

"You can get that kind of infection if you've broken a bone and it's protruding out of your skin."

"Geez, Doc, I don't have any broken bones sticking out of my body. I think we can eliminate that source. What else?" I asked rather facetiously.

"Another entry point, Jo-Ann, is through a lung infection."

"Well, Doc, I don't even have a cold nor any sniffles, so once again, I really do think we can rule that one out, too. Listen, Doc. I was very sick. Something caused a full blood infection. We've eliminated weepy battlefield wounds, broken bones, and severe lung infections. To me, what's left is that I have diverticular disease. Could the source be from my bowel, possibly something has burst? Seems to me we should be investigating my bowel as a possible source." I was pleading by this time.

"The hospital scanned you. You've had ultrasounds. The best in the business, in my opinion, reviewed the results. Are you feeling better?"

"Yes."

"Then continue taking your anti-inflammatory medication, and have a Merry Christmas." He ended our consultation. And, that was that.

Out of the Pan and into the Fire

The antibiotics administered at the hospital worked quite well and I had a really nice Christmas that year. But, this was not to last very long. By January, I was starting to feel ill, fatigued, and in pain again. There were never enough bathrooms for my needs. I continued through the months of February, March, and April. During this time my doctor took blood tests, white cell counts were very high, I was running a low-grade fever constantly now, and I was in a great deal of pain. There continued to never be enough bathrooms, and I was spending a lot of time in the ones I found. Gosh, do I have something to say to the toilet paper industry!

I was on a treadmill of illness, antibiotics, anti-inflammatory medication, blood tests, illness, and another round of antibiotics. You get the picture. By May of 2011, my body was becoming quite weakened so my very active lifestyle was now a thing of the past. I was beginning to realize that the only way to step off the treadmill would be to actually die. In my body, mind and soul I knew I could not go on much longer.

Is Anybody There? Can Anybody Hear Me?

May of 2011 found me attending another appointment with my doctor. "Geez, Doc, this is not normal. I'm so ill, and I don't even want to discuss with you what is coming out of me during my constant visits to the toilet. Don't you think I should be seeing some specialist? Doing the same thing over and over again and expecting different results, isn't that the definition of insanity? This is insane. I want to be referred to some kind of specialist. I'm sick, in pain, tired and I think I'm dying."

"I do believe we've run the course. I'll refer you to an Internal Specialist. You'll get a call from my office within the next few days."

If I hadn't been so sick, I would have done my version of the happy dance. Finally, we were doing something else. What would come of it I did not know, but anything was better than doing the same thing over and over and over again!

Yes, Virginia, There Is a Santa Claus

I was very fortunate regarding waiting time, and the Internal Specialist was able to see me June 1, 2011. We had a very interesting consultation. I had journaled my illness to that point with dates, times, and descriptions, all organized in duplicate. I handed him his copy to follow along with me, and he then allowed me to talk as he referred to his copy from time to time. He did not interrupt. He gave me the time I felt I needed, and all the while he jotted notes into his laptop computer.

When I finished sharing with him — some of which was peppered with some venting — he looked at me with his big brown eyes and said, "Mrs. Tremblay, we do know you have an inflammatory bowel disease, but I do think there is more to it. So, I am pulling together a team of five. Myself, yourself (as part of the team), a surgeon, a gastroenterologist, and your family doctor. Don't worry. We're going to figure this out. My only concern is that we may have up to a nine-month wait for you to see the gastroenterologist. But I'll do everything I can to expedite this."

It was at this time that I felt someone had actually listened to me, expected me to be part of the healing. Wow. I actually had a medical team in the making. Most of all, what I felt was hope again. Blessed hope. What a wonderful thing.

When I was growing up in Dartmouth, Nova Scotia in the 1960s, we had a nanny housekeeper. Mrs. Williams is descended from slaves that had made it to Canada. She lived in an area called Preston. As racism was rampant when the first groups of black people came to Nova Scotia, many all-black communities, villages and towns were set up. Most of these communities were located in a rural setting, one of which was East Preston.

Every day she came to work with a smile on her face. I don't remember a day without her wonderful smile. Her family and neighbours were hard-working folk, yet they always seemed to live on the edge of poverty. Many more seemed destitute. On Sundays, the residents of Preston would dress up in their most colourful and lovely Sunday finest, and head to church. There they would sing, sway to the music, dance in the aisles, and praise their God. This amazed me. How could they be so joyous? How could they be so colourful? How could they work so hard and receive so little in return?

One day, while sitting at the kitchen table with Mrs. Williams, I decided to satisfy my curiosity. "Mrs. Williams, you work really hard and I notice some people are not very nice to you. How can you always be so smiley?" I asked this with all the innocence of a young child.

She responded by saying, "Hope. It's all about hope, Jo-Ann. I live on hope. Hope nourishes me."

That was the day I began to understand the power of hope.

So, at least for the next while, as I waited to connect with my medical team, I knew I could live on hope, and that hope would nourish me. Not sure I had the fortitude of Mrs. Williams, her family and neighbours, but I sure was going to give it a try.

The illness progressed, and as promised, I received a call from a surgeon's office and was booked in to see him July 28. I then received a call from the gastroenterologist's office and I was booked for a July 20 appointment. I couldn't believe my ears. What was supposed to be an approximate nine-month waiting period had turned into only a nine-week wait. My doctor must have cashed in a few chips. I was so grateful. Hope continued to shine.

Unfortunately, the illness was moving along at a fast pace. I was very ill. I was now spending most of my days and evenings supine. I had lost a lot of weight. With no strength or body fat left, I was exhausted. July 1 came and my husband and I were invited to my sister and brother-in-law's cottage. I am an outdoor person, and being in the wilderness and sharing time with our beloved family was so tempting that although I was so ill, it was off to the cottage by the lake for us. I figured if I were going to die, there wouldn't be a better place to do it, nor better people to be the last folks I saw on this earth. We loved our four days at the cottage. I spent a lot of time in the outhouse with a beautiful view of the lake, developed a severe limp, but I had a wonderful time.

With a limp added to my list of symptoms, I could only

shake my head in confusion. On July 19, I received a call from the gastroenterologist's office and they were required to re-schedule my appointment from July 20 to the following Monday, July 25. Although it would be only five days, I queried myself: can I actually survive until Monday? Gosh, I don't know how I'm going to make it through the next five days. This is going to be such a big challenge, I really don't think I can keep going. My hope was fading.

Clean Underwear and Hair

Wednesday July 20 was the lowest of the low days for me. I was falling apart both physically and psychologically. As the day progressed, the pain in the core of my body intensified. I had very little energy, and I was giving up psychologically. Many times I found myself mulling over the thought, "I think I have to throw the towel in."

Wednesday evenings are special for us, it's the day of the week Johnny Vegas and his All-Star band perform. It's such a treat to hear our Beki sing. The fun and volume at Maxwell's is enough to wake the dead, it's all such a hoot. But not for me on that July 20. As the day continued, I was moving from bad to worse. With some encouragement, I convinced my husband Mark to go on his own to Maxwell's.

"I'm just going to lie in bed for the evening. Go. Have a good time. Say hello to Beki, Johnny and the band. Tell them to break a leg for me. Have a good time and I'll see you later." I waved goodbye.

With that, Mark left and I was alone lying in my bed, feeling broken and trying so very hard to find something positive to think about. The pain was intensifying, and it was becoming more and more difficult to lift myself up to go to the bathroom. The thought suddenly struck me: this is the worst I've ever felt in my life. I think, this is what an extreme situation feels like. I made my way to the bathroom for the, gosh, let's see — the 100th time today? And as I eliminated, I was also voiding brown urine.

Oh no. I think I'll have to go to hospital, there's something really wrong. My body is breaking! If I go to the hospital, I'm sure they'll keep me there. I've been so sick I've not had the energy to do a laundry. I can't go to the hospital without clean underwear. Isn't that one of the first lessons we learn from our mothers. Okay, I'll just throw my underwear in the washer.

Getting down the stairs to our laundry location was an excruciating trek. This was another indication to me that I was more ill than I had initially thought. Let's face it, I'd been so ill for so long, had endured incredible pain for years now, that I really didn't know where the line of extraordinary pain and you're-on-your-last-leg-kiddo started or ended.

There's a boiling frog story I have heard that seems to fit quite well for me at this time. The story is a widespread anecdote describing a frog slowly being boiled alive. The premise is that if a frog is placed in boiling water, it will jump out, but if it is placed in cold water that is slowly heated, it will not perceive the danger and will be cooked to death. The story is often used as a metaphor for the inability of people to react to significant changes that occur gradually, the upshot being that people should make themselves aware of gradual change lest they suffer eventual undesirable consequences.

Boiling frogs aside, my underwear was being washed in the machine, and so, my next thought was: Well, if I'm going to be in the hospital possibly for a while, I want to arrive there clean. I turned on the shower and had a devil of a time getting into it. Cleaned up and then in more pain than I can ever remember, I headed to the phone to call Mark at Maxwell's. Well, he was at the bar, the band was belting out their tunes, and he did not realize his cell phone was ringing.

Oh dear, I'll have to try to make it to the computer room and look up Maxwell's phone number online. OK, I'm here, wow the pain is so intense it's getting harder to think. Got their website, good, dial the number Jo-Ann, you can do it.

"Hello, yes. My name is Jo-Ann Tremblay. My husband, Mark, is at the bar upstairs. . . . Excuse me, I'm sorry what did you say? . . . Yes, I understand the Bistro is closed, but you see this is a family emergency. I need to inform my husband he needs to come home right now. Please speak with the bartender, Andy, upstairs. He's a friend and he knows my husband. He can get the message to him. But ensure you tell him he's to drive carefully, but get home as quick as possible. Thank you."

Good, I don't have to call an ambulance.

A moment later the phone rang and I answered. "Yes Mark, I'm not well at all. I need to go to hospital. Drive carefully."

By this time I no longer felt my body nor its parts, I was simply experiencing total and profound physical agony.

I was beginning to think I had waited too long. Throughout that evening my thinking had been that the worst of the pain and sickness would subside to a tolerable level. It had done so every time in the past few months. Tonight would be different, though. *Well, at least I'm wearing clean underwear, and my hair and body smell like a fresh orchid. I'm ready to live or die.*

Bon Voyage

Mark arrived, with suppressed panic in his eyes.

"Honey, they say we're going to have a storm tonight. Please go close the patio umbrella."

"Close the umbrella? To hell with the umbrella! We're off to the hospital!"

"No, please, Mark. I don't want the umbrella to break or blow away."

"I'm closing it," he replied and down the stairs he ran.

With the umbrella closed he returned to the room to collect me.

"Honey, I think they'll be keeping me. I grabbed some night clothes and dumped them on the floor there. I just couldn't get them packed. Could you please pack them into the overnight bag for me?"

"Geez, Jo-Ann," he stated with expletives as he grabbed some of the clothes on the floor and stuffed them — and I do mean stuffed them — into the bag.

In retrospect, I realize now that I was so ill and there was so much infection in my body that I was not really thinking straight. My brain was not functioning at its best. Not one of my stellar brain moments, to say the least. I like to be clean and I like to be organized, but this was a little extreme, even for me.

Mark helped me off the bed, and I was able to make it down the stairs, out the door, and into the car using my own legs, but with a great deal of help from Mark. Ottawa is often referred to as The Pothole Capital. Well, they're right! I felt every hole, dip, chip and crack in the street on the way to hospital.

Upon arrival, I of course needed to go to the bathroom, which I did. Moving from the wheelchair to the toilet was excruciatingly painful, and this took my last vestige of energy. By the time we arrived at the registration desk, I was simply going through the motions of breathing. The young lady took my blood pressure and it registered 54 over 38 and plummeting.

After a quick phone call to triage, she grabbed the wheelchair and raced down the hall, constantly asking "Are you still with me?"

I heard her and responded with "yes" each time.

Her voice seemed to be coming from the bottom of a barrel and it was getting fainter and fainter.

I was rushed into an emergency triage room, and the activity started. My earth angels disguised as nurses and a doctor, worked with me. I was stabilized to a certain extent — for the time being — and many questions and tests were conducted, which included another CT Scan. This type of scan is a computed tomography (CT) scan, which is an imaging method that uses X-rays to create cross-sectional pictures of a body. You lie down on a narrow table that slides into the centre of the scanner. Once you are inside the scanner, the machine's X-ray beam rotates around you. A computer creates separate images of the body area, called slices. These images can be stored, viewed on a monitor, or printed on film. Three-dimensional models of the body area can be created by stacking the slices together. You must be still during the exam because movement causes blurred images. You might be told to hold your breath for short periods of time.

As the CT Scan attendant tried to find a vein to administer the special dye, called contrast, to be delivered into the body before the test started (contrast helps certain areas show up better on the X-rays), my veins were actually imploding one by one. Hmm . . . I, at this point, assumed this was not good. Well, enough of the contrast dye did in fact enter my body and into the now-all-too-familiar machinery I slid.

After a number of hours, the doctor raced into my emergency room stall. "We found bubbles!"

"Cool," I thought. "I love bubbles. Wait a minute. Bubbles? What the heck are bubbles doing in my abdomen?"

"Not good, Mrs. Tremblay. What we do know right now is that you have peritonitis. We don't know the source yet, but you will be undergoing surgery. Arrangements are being made now."

My earth angel doctor helped us know that if I had arrived an hour later, I would probably not be alive at this point. His next concern was the three-and-a-half to four-hour surgery I had to undergo, and suggested that my husband and I say our goodbyes, as he was concerned with my weakened condition, that my chances of surviving the surgery were not good.

The rest of that night is a blur. I remember seeing my husband sitting on a chair with my overnight bag at his feet. I remember seeing him leave my curtained space from time to time with my overnight bag slung over his shoulder. I remember him holding my hand, smiling and whispering love messages, with my overnight bag placed carefully on the chair next to him. I remember lying in my bed in the hospital hallway with Mark by my side, kissing me, wishing me love, with my overnight bag hanging off of him. I knew my overnight bag was on strong shoulders and in good hands.

I made peace with my maker, whispered my love to Mark, and was wheeled into the operating theatre. It was not beyond me to know that this might be the last of my time on this beautiful and incredible planet. I thought of the many events, good and not so good, that I have endured. I thought of the grand and not-so-grand folks I had known, and those who shared my current life with me. I know that I am satisfied that I've done the best I could, that I've made mistakes, but that I've done good things, too. I've had unimaginable adventures. Who could ask for more? I'm ready for whatever comes.

But, before they put me under, before I was possibly taking my last breath, I decided that I was going to be very pleasant and chit chatty with the angels dressed in medical scrubs all around me, they, by this time, seeming too numerous to count. Let's face it, my life is now in their hands. I certainly want to impress upon them that I'm worth saving. Oh, the thoughts that go through one's mind when it's clouded with infection and the prospect of death.

I underwent the surgery to save my life. I survived — yay — and I emerged from the operating room with a very big change in how I am now going to live the rest of my life.

Positive stress, negative stress — stress no less. It's all in how you manage your energies. — Jo-Ann L. Tremblay

Wakey Wakey

Waking up in the recovery room is such a disorientating experience. "Well hello. You've sure kept us busy," said a blurry human form beside me. "It's about time you woke up. No, don't take that thing off, you've had a little trouble breathing. Your husband and son are waiting outside. I'll get your husband."

"Please ensure my son comes in also."

"We'll I'm not sure about that, dear. I'll go out and speak with your husband and take it from there."

"I don't understand. I want my son in here with me, as well. We need to see each other. We need to know we're both okay." Every fibre in my body screamed.

Gosh, what a blurry room, I can hardly see anything. Oh yeah. I'm in the recovery room. That's right. I've had surgery. Oh yes, now I get it.

"Hello again, Jo-Ann. Your husband and son are on their way. I'm sorry I didn't realize your son is an adult. I thought he was a child. That's why I had to check on him. I'm sure at 33 years old, he won't cause any disturbances — tee hee."

Seeing both my son, Richard, and my husband, Mark, was wonderful. I'm alive! I survived! They wore a smile on each of their faces, one with brown eyes and the other with blue ones. I could see how tired they both looked.

Things were not as blurry at this point. I also realized that they both had strained smiles, and knowing them both as well as I do, I thought there must be more to what has happened than I realize.

Anyone who has awakened from surgery knows how groggy the mind can be. I realized I would have to wait a little while to ask questions, to get a better grip, to attain an understanding of what has happened to me.

Once my vitals had improved, I was moved from recovery to my new bed that would be my home for the next ten days.

It was time to discuss pain management strategies, antibiotic drips, epidurals, potassium drips, and so on, and so on. My body had more needles and tubes connected to beeping machines than any one body should have. Draining tubes thrust deep into my abdominal region were hooked up to bags hanging off the side of my hospital bed. It was all pretty dramatic looking to me.

"What on earth has happened to me?" I asked my new nurse.

With the efficiency of a well-seasoned veteran of many post-op arrivals she replied, "Wait till the team arrives tomorrow. They'll explain everything to you. Just rest for now. You've been through a lot."

"Oh. OK."

Disturbing TRUTHS!

The following day, lying in bed in a morphine and epidural haze, I am roused when the team walks in. The General Hospital in Ottawa, Canada is a teaching hospital. Therefore, four of the eight-member team of doctors who had worked on me through the surgery the day before came and stood by my bed. With them was a gaggle of resident medical students. A good looking crew they were, and eager to explain to me how bad my situation had been, what had happened, and what amazing medical miracles they had performed.

I was stunned to say the least. "My descending bowel had multiple perforations?" Things had been very bad with my intestines. Hmm . . . Swiss cheese comes to mind.

"Let me get this straight: I had perforations throughout the sigmoid region of the colon. My abdominal region was filled with poisonous excrement and pus, organs were pushed out of place, and there were perforations into my urethra and vagina. And so, eight separate doctors, each with their own specialized expertise, repaired my body parts. Well, how wonderful of them," I said.

"Oh, you performed a Hartman's procedure. The sigmoid section — I know that one. It's the descending colon, right? — of my large bowel. It was removed. Part of my rectal stump was also removed. Oh. I see."

"Wait a minute! You said you had to perform a Hartman's procedure. I have a colostomy. OK, what the heck does all that mean?"

Outdoor Plumbing

"Sigmoid colostomy is a procedure when fecal diversion is required," stated the head of the team. "We have diverted the fecal stream from the rectum and anus. This was necessary to remove the area of diseased bowel. We removed a section of your descending bowel and rectum. The operation was necessary. Your bowel was diseased and perforated."

"OK. But what happened to me? What's going on? What am I supposed to do now?"

"We made an incision in your abdomen. We removed the diseased area of the bowel. We had to remove some of your rectal stump. We repaired your damaged urethra, and vagina, and we removed your appendix. And we've made a colostomy."

"Excuse me for not understanding, but what is a colostomy?"

"A colostomy is the end of the colon brought to the surface and stitched to the skin through a small cut in the abdomen. Fecal waste will now pass through the colostomy — it's called a stoma — and it will then be collected in a bag that sticks to the skin with special colostomy equipment. A prosthetic so to speak." And with a satisfied smile, the head guy of this interesting motley crew, simply ended the consultation with, "You have a colostomy."

"Well. My gosh. That explains everything. NOT!"

Brain Freeze

Okay, I'm alive. Check. I have tubes pumping stuff into me and some draining stuff out of me. Check. I'm so filled with drugs I seriously don't know up from down. Check. My body feels numb and weird. Check. I'm pooping into a bag that is attached to my abdomen near my belly button. Check. Oh my gosh. I'm pooping into a bag!

As I press the buzzer for the nurse I am near panic.

"Can I help you," she asks.

"Yes, well, apparently I have a bag attached to me. I'm pooping into the bag. Am I understanding right?"

"Yes, you're understanding."

"OK. So I'm pooping into a bag. How is that working for me? Will I have this for a short while or a long while? Do I have some kind of hole in me? What happens when the bag fills up? Where do I get bags?" And, the questions kept on floating up through my foggy brain. It was probably a blessing that my brain was foggy. I think I would have died on the spot from an anxiety-induced heart attack. Geez, it was all so weird.

"Mrs. Tremblay, all your questions will be answered in due time. You've been through a lot. Just lie back and relax. Your next goal is to start working on getting up. And then starting to walk. You're on a floor that is not used to handling this kind of recovery. All the beds are filled on that floor. They're the ones who handle your type of situation. Don't worry, though. We're with you here and we'll help you through it. Within the next few days, the resident ET nurse will be coming to see you for a consultation. She'll help you understand your colostomy. She'll instruct you on how to take care of your stoma, and so on. Do you need anything else?"

"No, I don't need anything right now, thanks."

Oh my gosh. Those drugs must be really something, I thought. The hospital is sending an extraterrestrial nurse to talk with me. Apparently aliens must be the experts in dealing with my stoma, whatever the heck that is. Not sure why they're so savvy about poop bags though. Well, I'll just have to wait and see this amazing being from out there somewhere who's got all the answers.

It took days before my Florence Night-in-Alien, arrived at my bedside. She looked quite normal (human-like) to me and was really quite sweet. My problem was, I was still on some heavy-duty pain management medication and most of what she was saying really wasn't reaching my brain. What was reaching, was awfully garbled. Maybe she should try her extraterrestrial mind-melding technique on me, some of her information might find its way to a more conscious place.

Eventually, she got through to me what an ET nurse is. It's an individual who specializes in enterostomal therapy. These professionals are knowledgeable experts in wound, ostomy, and continence care. They are Registered Nurses with advanced and specialized knowledge and clinical skills. From acute care hospitals, outpatient community clinics, long-term care and in independent practice, an ET nurse provides holistic assessment and management as an inter-professional team member to meet the needs of individuals/families with ostomies, acute and chronic wounds, and urinary and fecal continence problems.

My ET nurse was very informative and was committed to maximizing my self-care. Trouble was, when she lifted my hospital gown and showed me the equipment that was now attached to my abdomen, I was terrified, yet fascinated.

She explained that I had a stoma which is affectionately referred to as a "rose bud". Some rose bud! It was the remaining end of my intestine hanging out of my body, and very scary looking to me. I'll never look at a rose the same way again. Of course, it was newly created so it had stitches all around the base of the stoma. She discussed the various equipment I would now need. First, I required a flange that would be attached to my body by an adhesive. Protruding from this flange would be a specially constructed bag that snapped onto the flange.

"These bags are amazing," she continued.

Oh yeah, a poop bag is right up there with the Seven Wonders of the World. I kept my facetious thought to myself.

She then replaced my used poop bag with a fresh clean one, demonstrating to me how simple the procedure was.

"Oh yes, this works for me," I said as another facetious thought skittered through my brain.

This is when I realized I was having a real attitude

problem. I didn't want to even look at the equipment, let alone the stoma. Oh dear, this was curious as I realized my anxiety level was escalating. This is when the tears I had held back for over three years began to pour, and pour they did. If a person could cry blood, I would have lost a pint or two. I spent the days that followed in hospital crying quietly after my visitors had left my bedside, and I didn't stop the flow until my next round of visitors once again arrived. Mixed in with the outpouring of tears was a welling up of anger. In a 24-hour period, my emotions would swing from profoundly sad, intensely angry, determined to heal mustering up the energy to sit up and eventually walk again, and trying to be a helpful and easy-to-manage patient. (This latter for the medical staff and my family.) It was hard work, and I was completely exhausted.

At this point — let's face it — I had the time, and so decided to explore that thing called attitude. We're all born with an attitude, and it is further programmed and developed as we grow and experience. Attitude is a natural part of our human selves. Our attitudes will have an effect on our fulfillment level in life. Our attitude underlies all of our experiences and expressions. It is valuable to inventory our basic attitudes, and this is what I knew I needed to do. A success attitude is the drive to empower every act with the intent of fixing anything that is bungling up the hard work you're doing. A person's attitude is a great factor in gaining confidence and obtaining desired results. Our attitudes play an important role in how easy or difficult an experience will be. My ally throughout my whole life in good times and bad has always been my attitude. In order to put my finger on my attitude pulse I realized it was time to flip my eyes inward to my inner self and take stock of things. With the goal of helping myself, I decided that the first step I needed to do was to reach in and touch my feelings of gratitude. This was a good first step, and would certainly go a long way in correcting the course my attitude was taking at this juncture.

Letter of Gratitude

I am very fortunate that when I fell ill, many people offered to pray for me. The prayer groups grew over a very short time. I was assured by friends, family and neighbours that they were praying for me. Then, to my amazement, I was being contacted by people I didn't even know through short e-mails of encouragement, from across Canada and the United States. I call them my Prayer Village. A soul- and heart-felt thank you still radiates to each of them, their loving thoughts and prayers touched me in so many ways. Words alone can not express my gratitude. The act of a group of people focused on a goal, combined with the power that transcends and permeates all, is capable of accomplishing miracles.

My husband was a rock. I don't know what I would have done without him. Mark took care of me, organized my prescriptions, made meals, and stood by my side throughout my hospital stays — and in the beginning changed my ostomy flanges and pouches.

My son Richard was, and still is, my anchor, standing by my side throughout my hospital stays, helping in so many ways, including mommy-sitting me when Mark needed some time on his own, or phoning me with messages of love and keeping me up to date on his life with his amazing wife, Colleen, and our grandson, Evan.

Beki, one of my husband's daughters and who works at the hospital, took time from her lunch hours to drop by to visit me. She was truly wonderful.

My mother and father stood by my bedside as they supported Mark and Richard.

I had a long and challenging healing path ahead, but all in all I was doing okay, adjusting physically and psychologically to my new body. Each day, I was thankful for more life to live, and for the amazing people who made it worth living. I was stabilized and the crisis was over. I hoped. Looking back on it now, there were other circumstances when I just had to let go and let others come to rescue me. I can honestly say, it took the whole village to sustain me: my family, my friends, my neighbours, my doctors and nurses, my prayer village, and my support group. People have asked me, "How did you get through this ordeal so well?" And my reply, "I had help — lots of it."

PART 2

Know Yourself

As you travel the road of life, your self-concept is the pedal that controls your speed. — Jo-Ann L. Tremblay

Success lies in your ability to be the captain of your ship, and master of your destiny. — Jo-Ann L. Tremblay

Homeward Bound

After ten days, it was time to leave the security of the hospital and its knowing staff, and to come out to my new normal. I sure didn't feel ready, but it was time to get on with the healing process. By the way, due to the tubes coming into and out of my body, and the wound from the incision, and the like, not once did I use any of my clean underwear — nor my nighties — throughout my whole hospital stay. Mark pointed that out to me when he picked up my unopened overnight bag as we left the hospital. Oops . . .

Arrival back home was an interesting experience. With my husband Mark and my son Richard right there with me, I was gently deposited into my bed. Both Mark and Richard were amazing. They reviewed the documents sent home with me. They lined up the many medications. They began setting up my medication schedule. As I lay in bed feeling quite incapable of doing anything for myself, I could not but be amazed with my two caregivers. With some nerves beginning to wake up, I could feel the equipment attached to my abdomen and I worried as to how I was going to clean myself up, remove the used flange and bag.

I couldn't even sit up without a great deal of effort. Heavens! Surely I cannot expect my husband to have to do all of this for me.

We awaited the arrival of a health-care nurse scheduled to arrive within a couple of hours, and who would launch me on my amazing journey toward recovery. A PICC line (peripherally inserted central catheter) had been inserted into me while in hospital, to dispense a blend of four different antibiotics around the clock for about a month. This tube typically is inserted into the upper arm and advanced until the tip terminates in a large vein in the chest near the heart. It is used to obtain intravenous access. The antibiotic intravenous solutions were also scheduled to arrive from the Ontario Medical Supply (OMS) within a few hours. Various dressings for my wounds would also come from the OMS. It was time for a little rest before the show was to begin.

Ding dong went the doorbell and my intravenous solutions and boxes of wound-care supplies arrived. Richard and Mark carted the boxes upstairs to create a pharmaceutical dispensary in the corner of the bedroom.

Ding dong went the doorbell once again. My homecare nurse had arrived. Both Mark and Richard greeted her and led her upstairs to my bed where I was holding court. She had instructions to care for my six-inch abdominal wound, and to hook up my intravenous line. This consisted of an IV bag and a large and rather heavy box which housed the timing/dispensary mechanism that would slowly drip the fluid into my body via the PICC line over a 24-hour period. All of this was then placed in a canvas bag that had a handy transport strap. I named my IV equipment "Blooey" — not too original a name as the canvas bag was blue.

As the nurse prepared to examine my wound, to her surprise, she saw the colostomy equipment attached to my abdomen. "Oh my," she exclaimed. "I wasn't told you're an ostomate."

Great, I thought. *First of all what's an ostomate? Second, this is not starting very well!*

The nurse, being the professional she was, did not give much of an outward indication that this was a sticky situation for her. But I could tell that her mind was zooming all over the place.

Then, with a determined voice spiced with a light sense of humour, she spoke: "What supplies did the hospital send home with you? Let me see them. Not to worry, these things happen quite a lot." Her gentleness reassured me. "That's why we homecare nurses carry all forms and types of supplies in the trunks of our cars. I'll be right back."

With that, she rushed out the front door to her car. With two hands full of additional supplies, she was back in the bedroom. It was at this time that she placed a call to her headquarters to enlighten them that they were dealing with more than IV and wound care.

My caregivers, my advocates, and my protectors suddenly had that sinking feeling that there had been an administrative SNAFU at the hospital. Caregivers/advocates must not only pay attention to the doctors, nurses, and medications, as it turns out, it is also important that they pay particular attention to the administrative details. Now this is all a very demanding and complicated job. In most cases our advocates are not medically trained, and they do not necessarily know all of the administrative details required. They do not know what forms should be filled out, they don't necessarily know the pertinent information required for the proper completion of the forms, and all the while they are worried and concerned for their charges. How challenging is this? Let our experience provide an insight to caregivers: Do not take the administrative details for granted. Even with the best of know-how and intentions, SNAFUs happen. Pay close attention, scrutinize, and don't be shy to ask questions when dealing with forms and administrative details. It sure can save a lot of future frustration, as we found out at my homecoming, and then again, a month later.

With everyone now on the same page, and with a bedroom filled with medical supplies, a medicine cabinet shelf lined up with a variety of pain management medications and other pills to counter some of the side effects of the pain medications, Blooey and I settled into a strange, and at times harsh, journey to recovery. The doctors had warned me that from beginning to end I would be looking at a year-long recovery. Needless to say, I was not going to push myself hard at this point.

My days were filled with Mark's administering scheduled medications every four hours around the clock. Every day I awaited my health-care nurses. It was such a delight when they arrived. I was taken care of by a team of four nurses, each one a professional with that personal touch. They were incredible and I enjoyed their administrations and delightful personalities. They were a godsend. Mark, Richard and I felt a high degree of confidence knowing my nurses were with us.

Oh yes! An "ostomate" is a person who has an ostomy. I now had a new title.

Ka-Blooey

Blooey proved to be an interesting buddy. First, the intravenous bag was quite heavy (in my weakened state). Of course, the whole mechanism was tethered to a vein in my upper right arm. From there, the life-preserving medication flowed through me to a main vein, into the heart that then carried it to all parts of my body. Blooey had a nifty over-the-arm strap that I would put over my shoulder when I got out of bed and moved around, but I was still limited to the bedroom and bathroom. Not being used to Blooey, and then, of course, with the drugs that fuzzed up my brain, numerous times I simply started to get up forgetting to bring the equipment with me, when all of a sudden Blooey would not budge. The vision of an animal running to the end of its rope and flipping over came to mind. I lost count as to how many times I did this. Geez, that was smart!

Baby Steps

As each day passed, I gained more strength and although my world was still very small, I began to expand my horizons. Slowly, I started navigating the stairs. This would bring me from the upstairs to the main floor, and then to another set that I navigated to the TV room in the basement family room. During this time, family and friends sent food CARE packages to us, from homemade soups, yummy chicken pies, tourtières, pâté chinois, and other wonderful meals. (Special thanks went to my mom for her goodies, Nola for the chicken and meat pies — they were the best — and Betty's soup warmed my bones. Many others were there for us, too.)

Showers Are Always Interesting

The last shower I took before surgery was on July 20, under dire circumstances. Throughout my hospital stay, I was not permitted to shower. I was reduced to hand washing strategic spots only. As I was not very dexterous due to intravenous lines running into my hand, washing required some very interesting body contortions. I must admit, I was quite amazed with myself.

Of course, I was unable to wash my hair at this time, either. Even when I was on my way to losing my life I had been intent on arriving clean, so you can imagine how uncomfortable I was by this point. My last hair wash had been when I was in hospital. One of the nurses had realized this was a personal hygiene calamity for me, and had offered me a new and amazing method of cleaning hair without using water. It looks like a shower cap, and is placed over the head to the hairline. Then, with vigorous massaging, a cleansing chemical is released which cleans the patient's hair. *Wow! What will they think of next!* I felt a little more human when we finished, and I am grateful for this lovely lady and her amazing magic hair tonic.

It would be September 2011 before I was finally able to take a full shower. Because of the intravenous line and surgical wound, immersion in water was not permitted. As time passed and as I grew stronger, Mark (my guardian angel), washed my hair in the kitchen. As I stood in front of the sink, he would gently scrub my hair, rinse, give my hair a second wash, and then add a dab of conditioner, wait a moment, and then rinse again. Amazing how resourceful we can be when push comes to shove.

As I grew stronger in the days that followed, I was able to wash my own hair at the sink. I noticed during these times that large amounts of hair were coming out of my head and getting entangled around my fingers. *Oh great, I'm going bald now too.* As I had been so ill and of course given so much medication, I realized it had taken its toll, and hair loss would just have to be a fact of life for me. *Hmm . . . Better to have a bag, bald and scarred up, than be in a bag,* ran through my mind on more than one occasion.

Our beliefs determine our thoughts, behaviours, and actions; they in turn determine our outcomes. — Jo-Ann L. Tremblay

Attitude Is Everything

By now, my whole self and life was in transition physically, emotionally, mentally and in spirit. It was difficult to even imagine what was around the corner for me. I barely knew the right questions to ask or the best adjustments to make. The uncertainty I was experiencing could lead me in different directions: I could succumb to anxiety and be overwhelmed, or I could rise to the occasion with a good attitude sprinkled with courage. It was thinking time again.

My world continued to expand. I could now navigate the stairs — although slowly and in a strange crawling motion — but I was able to go up and go down. This was exciting! With Blooey over my shoulder, I began to sit out on our patio and enjoy the summer filled with breezes, songbirds, grass, trees, and little bugs. I was glad to be alive and to have a second chance at life. Those were the positive-thought moments. But then there were the dark-thought moments. The pendulum would swing from one extreme to the other. As I sat in the warm sunshine, I would often feel cold to the bone. Bewilderment took over on an almost daily basis. That I was nearing a precipice over which I might fall to my death, came often. My thoughts and feelings would scatter from: *I was an hour from death in July. Surgery saved my life. God I'm in so much pain. I poop in a bag. What has all of this done to my future health prospects? Damn it, I do have a second chance here, so onwards and upwards!*

It was a time of tumult. Perhaps I was half mad with stress? Sometimes I wonder how I managed to get through it all. I guess we are more resilient than we give ourselves credit for. We never know just how tough we are until circumstances force it from us.

One Day, One Moment, One Breath at a Time

In 2008, when my illness and pain had become chronic, there were times when I was only able to take life one day at a time. Through the years that followed, I was eventually reduced to coping with my body and life one moment at a time. During these times, I often found myself searching, trying to find any reason, any excuse, to have a positive attitude, a positive outlook. I, of course, could find many. I am very fortunate to be blessed in so many ways. But as time advanced along with the illness, I realized that I could not go forward on positive thoughts alone. In fact, I realized that I was not being totally honest with myself in thinking I was being positive while knowing in my heart that I was downright miserable. My mind was in a push-me-pull-me mode. I endured the physical pain as I was drowning in an emotional quagmire. I was sick, angry, and fighting for my quality of life.

As the illness progressed, I arrived at the realization that I was taking life one breath at a time now. It was becoming more and more challenging to remain honestly positive so I decided there must be another way. I could try to talk myself into "positive thinking" until I was blue in the face, but in reality there came the understanding that this approach, this life tool, was not working for me anymore. It was not the appropriate tool for this circumstance. It was not real. It was a mask. It was dishonest. It was downright denial. I needed to step down into the depths of my current reality with eyes wide open. Be truthful with myself. I had to look the monster of my illness and my predicament in the eye, with full awareness.

Aha! Awareness. That's the ticket! I began to insert awareness as a coping tool, rather than positive thinking more often than not. In my attempts to simply be aware in the very breaths I took, I used this tool to help develop a deeper understanding of my individuality and the many aspects of myself, my illness, and the life all around me. With full awareness focused and interwoven into each breath, I eventually became sensitive to the truths I was operating from, those I was expressing, and the true realities of my situation. It was honesty, not a fantasy in all its wonder and all of its ugliness. A value-added bonus to this approach was an immersion into the fullness of breath. With every inhale and exhale I realized that time expanded on occasion to the place of forever. I was beyond positive thinking and had arrived at a place where I realized that any one of us can die at any time. It could be today, it could be tomorrow, or in twenty years from now — who really knows? The only thing that *is* true is that the "now", the "present", is the reality that exist. It is up to us to put as much into and receive as much as possible from that breath, that moment, that day. I was hurting in all ways possible, so it was hard to see a positive future, but it was easy to immerse into my breath and explore the depths, wonders, and potentials a breath can hold. Like a string of pearls, my string of breaths encircled me with the hope and the strength that life — at least for the moment — continued.

I live in awareness because I could die today, tomorrow, or in twenty years from now. I really don't know. Awareness as a tool works for all times, circumstances and situations during the course of a lifetime. Positive thinking is a great tool, one that is appropriate when we are working hard and anticipating a successful outcome. Positive thinking is a tool of great usefulness, but it is not the only tool in our personal and professional toolbox.

Sitting on my patio on those warm summer days during my recovery, I found myself looking back, and looking forward. Awareness is a valuable tool I will use quite regularly and continue to hone as my life continues to unfold.

More Deep Thoughts

When the "How are you?" question pops up since the surgery, my impulse is to run a million miles away faster than the speed of light, and this is quite irresistible. I don't want to be the sum total of my tragedy. It has been difficult, but I'm getting over it. I am moving on. I don't want to talk grief and I don't want to talk illness. And the last thing I want to share with others is all the weird physical things that have happened and that are continuing to happen to me. Despite all the physical changes and issues at this time, I am still a fit person. I don't sound like one, though, if I talk with people. "No, I don't want to talk about how I am. I'm fine thanks," is all I want to say. But when I do shorten my response, people will then ask, "I mean, how are you, really?" I guess as they say, what doesn't kill you makes you stronger?

Grapefruit

Step by step, I began to take control of my ostomy care. I must say in the beginning it took a great deal of courage on my part to even look at my stoma. There is just something unnatural about an intestine protruding from one's abdomen. I was repulsed by the whole idea. Let's just say I had a lot of work to do to change my attitude.

Then one day I noticed that I had a grapefruit-sized bulge under my stoma. I had noticed a small protrusion in the weeks before, but now it was a very noticeable bulge. *Geez, what is it? What's wrong with me, now? I'm scared, what can it be?*

I started making phone calls beginning with my surgeon. She was unable to call me back. Her assistant suggested I call my family doctor. I called him. He was on holidays. I called Home Care, the organization from which my amazing home-care nurses worked for. They would have an ET nurse call me back. I waited. No phone call came fast enough for me. It was a full week before the ET nurse called me. Although I did not feel physically any different than I had the day before, I was terribly frightened of what the bulge might mean. I called the phone numbers of various ostomy clinics that were printed in some of the material sent home with me when I was discharged but unfortunately, I was told that I would have to wait until someone could call me back to make an appointment. Now it must be understood that not having experienced an ostomy, being a newbie at this, I had no idea if the bulge was an emergency situation or not.

I then found the phone number for the United Ostomy Support Group of Ottawa (affiliated member of United Ostomy Association of Canada). Once again, I was presented with another earth angel. Within minutes of placing a call to their emergency line, a volunteer called me back. I described my bulge to the gentleman. He asked me a number of relevant questions. He, of course, was a fellow ostomate volunteer and his reassuring voice relaxed my jagged nerves. His thought was that it is probably a "parastomal hernia", and recommended I call my doctor and make an appointment. If I were to feel any strange pains, blockages or what-have-you in the meantime, he urged me to go to Emergency immediately.

Groping in the Dark

This bulge was the beginning of the realization that very few medical people have either the desire or the expertise to work with ostomies and stomas, at least in my part of the world. The good and bad news was: I was developing a "parastomal hernia", I was not in deep trouble, and my recovery would continue.

A parastomal hernia is a weakness, split, or other defect in the muscle wall of the abdomen and which allows the abdominal contents (usually a part of the intestine such as the small bowel, colon, etc.) to bulge out. When a stoma is created, the bowel is brought to the surface of the abdomen and must pass through the muscles of the abdominal wall via an artificially created split. This split becomes a site of weakness. In an ideal situation, the abdominal wall muscles fit snugly around the stoma opening. However, sometimes the muscles will come away from the edges of the stoma thus creating a parastomal hernia in the area of the abdominal wall near the stoma where there is no muscle. The resulting weakness, or gap, means that every time one strains, coughs, sneezes, or even stands, the area of the abdomen next to the stoma bulges.

Without pointing any fingers, there were many situations and concerns that could or would not be answered by my various physicians. Mark and I felt that so often we were either hung out to dry or were sent groping our way through a dark forest. It was challenging, and frankly, we were often quite worried, not knowing if something I was experiencing was par for the course as far as ostomies were concerned, or that I had something really bad happening to me.

The Internet is amazing. We started a search and found out that parastomal hernias occur in approximately 20–50% of patients with stomas. Over the long term, the possible chance of having a parastomal hernia develop at some point becomes an inevitable one. Exercises to strengthen the abdominal muscles can be encouraged before surgery. Stoma-care nurses play a vital role in educating patients that may help reduce the incidence of developing a parastomal hernia.

Possibly because my surgery was an emergency situation and was not planned, I was never made aware of the possibility of developing a parastomal hernia, nor was I made aware that there are some preventive measures for the ostomate. I am surprised that neither the physicians nor the ET professionals in hospital had informed me of this potential complication.

I have since learned that for those folks who know they will be undergoing colostomy surgery, there are some abdominal exercises that can be done to strengthen the abdominal muscles before the surgery happens. It is also very important for an ostomate to wear an abdominal support belt while undertaking heavy lifting and heavy work for at least one year postoperatively.

In my situation, I did not lift anything heavy nor do any heavy work. It was simply that a parastomal hernia is a frequent difficulty for patients with stomas. I do wish we had known about this complication from the beginning. We would have acquired a hernia belt very quickly, and I would have worn it at all times with the exception of overnight sleep.

As it turned out, I was diagnosed with a parastomal hernia complication so we began to explore the Internet to find the best belt for me. After researching many hernia belt manufacturers, we then called the Ostomy Care and Supply Centre in New Westminster, Canada and spoke with the ET nurse/owner of the company. I discussed my situation and she was at once incredibly informative and helpful. She ordered two different styles of belts for me and had them shipped. Although I would rather not have to wear my hernia belts, especially in the heat of the summer, I know they are a must for me. Surgical repair will be explored in the more distant future.

What Else Can Go Wrong?

As though my body decided that everything I had been going through in the previous four years was not enough, I developed what we call "episodes". These episodes would at times be mild and at other times, they were close to being catastrophic.

One late afternoon, I was sitting out on our patio relaxing while Mark was working at the barbecue, grilling our dinner. I noticed strange things happening in my body. I felt like an accordion inside me had been stretched out and then one end of it had been let go of, so that everything inside me was collapsing and being crushed. It was not as though I felt dizzy and thought I would pass out. No, it was as though everything inside, all of my organs, were squeezing together.

I said, "Something's wrong with my body."

After Mark had placed me on the floor, he took my blood pressure. It was 52 over 36. Time to call the ambulance!

The paramedics arrived, and thankfully I had started to feel a bit better. The worst had gone by and now I was, as I put it, "coming back". After taking my vitals, their recommendation was to bring me to hospital immediately. *Wow! I get to ride in the ambulance this time. Cool.*

After I arrived at hospital, my vitals became more and more normal as the minutes went by. Mark, Richard, paramedics and the other poor souls that had been brought to the Emergency by ambulance that evening had a "hospital hallway party". Again, I must mention that the Ottawa paramedics and the General Hospital ER nurses were outstanding. All professionals with that personal touch.

It would be months, there would be visits to cardiologists, and a number of other emergency hospital crises would occur before I could actually begin predicting, through subtle physical symptoms, when I would next be at risk for another full-blown episode. Meanwhile, the doctors had no label for this medical issue and called it a mystery.

Oh, no. Not that word again! I'm starting to feel like the most mysterious lady in the world. The statement the doctor in 2010 made: "You're weird and God hates you" has skittered through my mind many times over.

The Mystery Solved — I Think

While attending a United Ostomy Association–National Capital Region meeting, at one point during the evening I was talking with the president of the Chapter when all of a sudden I began to experience that crushing feeling again. I started to sweat and felt very heated. He noticed this physical change immediately and directed me to a chair. Once I was seated, he asked me to describe my symptoms. As I did, he nodded his head in understanding with each symptom I shared. As it turned out, it was one of the milder episodes, thank goodness. The milder episodes can occur up to five times a day for me. Then, for no apparent reason, I will not experience them for a week or more. The more critical episodes seem to occur on average about once every four weeks. All this is to say that there is no pattern. For the milder episodes, there are no symptoms of what is about to happen until I'm actually experiencing the episode. Unnerving.

As my body calmed down that evening, he was able to help me understand that he, too, experienced episodes that were quite similar in nature to mine. In his case, his white cell count elevated. Interestingly, the blood tests I had undergone a couple of weeks before the meeting indicated that my white cell count, too, was elevated. He explained to me that in his case, it was realized that what remained of his colon was in fact not absorbing nutrients as it would have if he'd had a fully functioning large bowel. When this happens, the body automatically sends out white blood cells as it believes there is something wrong. White blood cells are the soldiers of our body. Like an army patrol, they travel through our blood stream looking for any invaders, ready to fend them off. This is what happens when we are fighting an infection, for example. Nifty little guys they are. When this occurs, we experience a drop in red blood cells as their job is to carry oxygen and nutrients through the body. The thing was, his body was being tricked to a certain extent. In reality, what it was for him was that what remained of his intestines were at times unable to absorb, or at other times inadequately absorb, the required amount of enzymes and minerals, etc. to maintain good functioning. The removal of part or all of the bowel is an amputation. It once had a job, now it's gone. What is left of the bowel will continue doing its work, and will even attempt to compensate for what has been lost, but it's a tall order. The bottom line for his condition was: when his intestines were unable to absorb an adequate amount of minerals, salts, etc., his body would go into crisis mode as it tried to deal with the situation, and all heck would break loose.

Basically, the intestinal tract comprises the stomach, the small intestine, and the large intestine or colon. Alcohol, some medications, and simple carbohydrates are absorbed directly from the stomach. From there, each section of the intestine is responsible for the absorption of a particular nutritional element.

The intestine seems to adapt to surgery and resections. However, the loss of the distal ileum and colon can affect nutritional absorption. Changes in nutritional absorption have been found to cause any number of health-related concerns. From my research, I understand that due to the anatomy of the intestine, there are affects on mineral and bile salt absorption, and on electrolytes, and so there are some latent deficiencies of essential vitamins and minerals. In addition, because the intestinal function is compromised, hydration becomes much more important for ostomates than for the average person.

The president shared a few of his tips with me. He said that when an episode begins to occur, to sit down immediately. It doesn't matter where I am or what I'm doing, sit down and relax. Carry a sports drink, and consume it. Sports drinks are filled with salts, potassium, etc., so this will flood the body with the nutrients that it is lacking at that particular moment. He suggested that I make an appointment with a blood doctor to have a full and proper blood analysis.

Although at this time we do not know yet definitively what my "mystery" health issue is, we are investigating the possibility that I am not absorbing certain enzymes or other nutrients. This part of the journey is still being explored with my physicians.

Supply And Demand

In the event that all of this wasn't enough, five months after the surgery, my parastomal hernia had grown to the size of a honeydew melon. It was time to buy new pieces of clothing to add to my wardrobe. I have always been quite slim, and I still am, so now I am slim with a melon-sized bulge on the left side of my abdomen. Not too easy to camouflage so I decided to hone my fashion sense and visit a few maternity shops. Quite the conversations I have had with store employees when, at the age of plus 55, I'm looking at styles in a maternity shop.

With my ever-expanding hernia horizons, fitting the best ostomy equipment has been a nightmare. To add to this change, my stoma is very active. It will prolapse (elongate) from about 2½ inches long, or shrink to a concave spot below my abdominal wall. These ins and outs will occur many times during the course of a day. *Geez, what equipment is best fitting for me?* During one visit to an ET nurse, I saw that she was concerned about the length of the stoma prolapse and recommended that I not use a convexity wafer as part of my equipment — this could be what was exacerbating the prolapse. My stoma was really sticking out that day, just hanging around, trying to look cool, I guess. I tried this. Well, it was all about breach. And, I'm not referring to a whale jumping out of water. Some of my appliances lasted only a few hours. Ostomy equipment is costly, and my breaches were getting very expensive for me. I visited another ET nurse and on this visit, my stoma was concave, a shy little one simply peeking out from the inside. She recommended that I wear a convexity wafer because when the stoma retracted to concave, the normal flange without convexity would not be a sufficient barrier. All this is to say, when my stoma — for whatever reason — retracts almost all the way in, the flow from my stoma can actually seep out underneath the appliance and its barriers. (This is when a nice brown spot on my outer clothing can appear.) There are many appliance designs to suit all body and stomal types. Some folks can wear an appliance that is flush with the skin, and others require convexity. A convex appliance simply means there is an outward curve which is designed to apply a form of direct pressure to the immediate peristomal skin, the idea being to promote a good seal between the ostomy pouching system and the skin.

OK, let's get this straight: I should wear convexity, and I shouldn't wear convexity. Now, isn't that a conundrum? Well, everybody is unique, and it certainly is a challenge for the ostomy industry to produce products that will work for all body types and stomas. It is equally challenging for the ostomate to select the best equipment for his or her needs.

I have been impressed with all of the ostomy appliance companies. They have ET nurses on staff who specialize in ostomy care, equipment, and in the company's various products. You need only call them and they will suggest products that may suit your situation. They will then mail samples. This has been so helpful for me. As I said, the cost of equipment is high, and with the use of samples, I have been able to explore and decide on the equipment that best suits my particular anatomy and requirements.

The fact remains for me, I have a very active stoma, and combined with a large hernia, it's all a challenge.

So, I'm half pregnant in appearance (five months on the left side) and my stoma seems to be doing the limbo. Oh. And by the way, my hair is still falling out. Hmm. My new normal is a strange one indeed.

The Things Friends Will Do for You — Thank You, Fran!

As the parastomal hernia increased in size, I realized I should be wearing reinforced underwear, and more specifically, a hernia belt. The underwear and/or belt provide some measure of support. I decided to start off with the underwear. Finding and purchasing the underwear was rather simple. Of course they do not come with a handy dandy reinforced hole in the most strategic location that will allow my equipment to be readily accessible and which would also not put undue pressure on my stoma. An ostomate is essentially incontinent, so clothing apparel must take into account that there might be a flow at any given time, and that flow must not be restrained or blocked in any way.

As I am unable to sew a button on straight, I realized I would need someone with the skills to design and sew a reinforced opening in the front of my reinforced underwear to accommodate my stoma and equipment all the while ensuring that the elastic quality of the underwear was not compromised.

As luck would have it, a dear friend of mine called me to say hello. During the course of our conversation I mentioned my hernia and underwear dilemma. She immediately offered to give it try. Besides being a giving and wonderful person, Fran is very creative, talented and an amazing seamstress. I jumped at the opportunity. As she and her husband live in their beautiful lake home in the wilderness, about a two-hour drive north of us, an invitation for a visit was offered.

What fun! A few days in paradise with wonderful friends, and new underwear. It doesn't get better then that!

Upon arrival, Fran scrutinized my stoma and equipment placement, measured and then measured some more. We poured a glass of wine and the creativity began. Taking one of her husband's old underwear, she removed the thick elastic waistband. She then took a pair of her own old underwear (she is frugal and didn't want to waste any one of my brand new pairs) as she went about designing the prototype.

Fran worked her haute pooture magic. She sewed with extreme attention to detail that only an expert seamstress can. It was time-consuming as she applied machine and hand-executed techniques. It took three days for the 4 pairs of underwear with their strategically placed reinforced circle openings made specifically to my measurements and body stance. When she had finished them, I admired my elegant haute pooture undergarments. Fran had even attached a specially embroidered teddy bear sporting a big smile upon his brown face at the side of one of my newly created panties. Now that's cute.

It always amazes me what friends will do for friends.

Stoma Naming Celebration

As my husband affectionately tells me "You're my little semicolon," for the rest of my life I will sport my colostomy, so it came time to make friends with it, to give it a name.

"I am really doing my best to accept this colostomy," I told Mark over a cocktail one evening. "I want to give my stoma a name. Since you have to live with it, and you're so good at naming things, what are your name suggestions?"

"Hmm. Percy! Percy comes to mind. Not sure why, but it does."

"Percy . . ." I rolled this name across my tongue as I looked down at my abdomen. "Percy. The good news is that we don't know anyone with the name Percy, so we won't be insulting them. Hmm. Percy is an interesting name. Percy is a good code name in that if I'm having any issues, I can simply state Percy is having a problem, and you'll discreetly know. Yep, Percy's a good name."

I went upstairs to the computer to research the name Percy. Percy name origin: Old English for "pierce the hedge". How brilliant is that? Time to have another drink and toast Percy. Let's face it, he keeps me alive. He gave me another chance at life. He's my hero.

And so it was the beginning of a lifelong respect and acceptance of my colostomy.

PART 3

The Adventures of Percy & Me

Celebrate the amazing person you are and experience the most thrilling journey of a lifetime. — Jo-Ann L. Tremblay

The power in each individual comes from all of us, and the power of all of us comes from each individual. — Jo-Ann L. Tremblay

The Good, the Bad & the Funny

Living with an ostomy has its ups, downs and all-arounds. It seems as though every week there was something good, something bad, and something humorous about living with Percy. I have always enjoyed a healthy sense of humour, and I seemed to consistently give myself a daily dose of reasons to laugh at myself and life under my old circumstances. In spite of myself, now that my ostomy had been created, the reasons for laughing at myself and life increased by many.

Percy's Coming-Out

We announced Percy's new name to our family and friends. From that day forward, the phone would ring, and "Hey, how's Percy?" the voice on the other end would ask. A friend would arrive. "How's Percy hanging?" they would ask in all seriousness.

This has been wonderful for me, for family and our friends. It has provided an opportunity for inquiry whereby I can share Percy's issues (or non-issues) as I choose, while still feeling healthy and vibrant in the rest of my body and life — although, I must admit, at times I am a little jealous of Percy's taking front stage. On the other hand, if it's been a particularly difficult day with digestion, equipment or whatever colostomy-related problems du jour, I can take it out on Percy My Little Pooper, which enables me to detach from the situation. This has been very empowering. Each of us cannot always control what happens to us, but we can control our attitudes. We are masters of ourselves, our lives, and how we adjust to the changes that arise in the course of a lifetime. We can disallow change to master us!

Cool Dudes & Dudettes: the United Ostomy Association

After the United Ostomy Support Group volunteer had so generously returned my call when I had inquired about the then-grapefruit-sized lump, and with the lack of knowledge out there in stoma world, I realized I needed to know more about this organization.

People with ostomies do not have to endure alone. There are many issues that arise with an ostomy, with being an ostomate, with being the caregiver of an ostomate, and there is a need for support. Over the years, there has been an evolution of organizations to educate, assist and empower persons with ostomies. The United Ostomy Support Group is affiliated with the United Ostomy Association of Canada (UOAC). This organization has been in place for many years working toward a common goal in supporting the needs of persons with ostomies, needs that include encouragement, emotional support, empowerment, and education.

The support group is a volunteer-run charitable organization dedicated to helping all persons, including families and caregivers, who have been affected by ostomy surgery. Their mission is to provide practical support and encouragement to all ostomates by visiting them at home or in hospital, by holding monthly meetings, by providing an assistance hotline, and through a monthly newsletter, outreach programs, sponsorship for an ostomate child to attend summer camp, educational seminars/training programs, and operating a lending library of ostomy literature.

I cannot say enough about these really cool dudes and dudettes. I have learned so much and the camaraderie is priceless.

Nerves & Nightmares

During my healing journey, from time to time I experienced excruciating pain that often hit an 8 on the 0 to 10 scale. When these pains in various locations in my abdomen occurred, I would be unable to stand up straight. At times, I would have to lie down on the bed and ride it out. On other occasions, the pain would last twenty-four hours, and at other times up to forty-eight hours. As I understand pain to be my friend (pain helps us know something is wrong), initially I was quite worried that the sensation of pain was trying to tell me something. A visit to the doctor helped me understand what occurs during these incidences.

As it turns out, many nerves must be severed during the type of surgery that will eventually produce an ostomy. There is also the potential of damage caused by an illness itself whether it is cancer, diverticular disease, or a host of other diseases a patient might have experienced and which has caused the need for surgery in the first place. Simply, there can be a lot of collateral damage.

In my case, during the times of the excruciating pain, it was determined that the basic issue was that another set of nerves were waking up — so to speak — from the disease and surgery trauma. They were now either becoming active or they had generated new branches and were going online, and so on. Those poor little nerves were waking up from a nightmare and sending wild messages that translated into pain. At other times, I would experience tremors, odd vibrations, and so on. The good news is that the nerves eventually realized "Aha! I've got it. We're okay." When I understood this situation, my anxiety lessened. So now, when I feel this pain, I remain calm, lie down, rest, endure, and wait it out for the twenty-four to forty-eight hours.

It's a disturbing peace of mind, but a peace of mind no less.

Sphincter Spectre

I would just like to say that some of us have to endure another interesting phenomenon associated with ostomy surgery. It's called Phantom Rectal Sensation. Good grief! I get to experience this amazing phenomenon as well? Phantom rectal sensation is similar to the phantom limb sensation of amputees who have the sensation that their removed limb is still there. As it turns out, it is normal for an ostomate to feel as if they need to evacuate through the rectum even though it is now non-functioning. Research states that this can occur for years after surgery. If the rectum has not been removed, one may also have this feeling and may pass mucus when sitting on the toilet. *Oh, this sounds like fun!* Some who have had their rectum removed say that the feeling is relieved somewhat by sitting on the toilet and acting as if an evacuation is taking place. I think at this point I've earned, at the very least, a Gemini Award nomination for Best Comedy Program or Series for toilet antics.

A Doctor's Concern

It was the first visit with my specialist since the emergency bowel surgery. Being the concerned physician he is, he knew my physical condition but was unsure as to where my emotional condition was at, and so, with an optimistic demeanour he asked: "Off the top of your head, from the tip of your tongue, can you tell me one good thing about your colostomy?"

My immediate response: "I haven't had to wipe my butt since July 21, 2011."

He sat motionless for about two seconds, then we both burst out laughing.

Flu and Chronic Conditions

Arriving at the flu clinic in our community, I filled out the forms, stood in line, and then was directed to one of the many nurses giving shots to the multitude. A very sweet middle-aged woman sat ready to receive me, and upon my arriving at her station, she asked: "Do you have any chronic illnesses?"

I sat for a few seconds trying to figure out if a permanent colostomy would be considered a chronic illness. I then said, well I have a colostomy, does that fit into the chronic category?

Then with an oh-my-gosh-you-poor-thing look on her face which was reflected in her voice she asked, "How is it working for you?"

"It's okay. In fact it's working quite fine as we speak."

After a few seconds of silence, a wide smile crossed her face and she chuckled and asked me to fold up the sleeve of my sweater for the shot.

Like the archer, you need a target to aim for; if not, you will shoot an arrow into the air and know not where it will land.
— Jo-Ann L. Tremblay

Stepping Out

Two months after my lifesaving surgery, and still very early into my recovery, our nephew and his beautiful fiancée were to be married. I must say I was filled with many conflicting thoughts and emotions. It would be my first time journeying out from the safety of my home as an ostomate. I was really not very strong, my PICC intravenous line had been removed by now and I was having Blooey separation anxiety. Attending a wedding would be a very ambitious goal for me, and I was not sure I was ready.

Ms. Bean Goes to a Wedding

My first time out in the big world since the surgery, my body had a new way of operating, and I was a greenhorn. Before leaving home, I had packed my courage and a carry bag filled with ostomy supplies. Mark loaded the wheelchair into the trunk of the car, me into the passenger seat, and my first adventure began.

Arriving at the venue, we settled ourselves in the tent waiting for the ceremony to begin. It registered 30 degrees Celsius (86°F) as the guests filed in and were seated. Within moments, the first of the beautiful bridesmaids walked over the little bridge and entered the tent. It was at this time I felt a "pop" on my abdomen and alarm bells began to go off throughout my body. *It couldn't be. No. Surely it was only a . . . a . . . ?*

Feeling very silly, and as discreetly as possible knowing the folks around me had eyes only for the bridesmaids, I reached under my waistband, slid my hand down my pants, and sure enough an ostomate's worst nightmare had begun. The adhesive that holds the flange had separated from the skin. There are various appliance designs — the one I use has two pieces to it (a flange and a bag), the flange is the part that adheres to your body. The bag snaps onto the wafer and collects the output from the stoma. There I was, on my first foray into the big world as an ostomate, all nestled in my wheelchair, and as Murphy's Law would have it, I was in the middle of my first equipment malfunction. My flange was threatening to pop completely off, and the bride had just stepped off the bridge and was now heading to the front of the tent where her groom awaited her. Their new life together was just about to begin and I was on poop alert.

The warm day started to feel even warmer, and all the while I was now simultaneously experiencing shivers and sweats. The shock of it all was getting to me. I glanced at the bride and groom sharing their vows, and then down to the front of me, hoping no brown spot would appear. The ceremony was beautiful and a perfect combination of not too long and not too short, a blessing for my predicament, indeed. It was a very busy ceremony for me. First, my joy of sharing in this special day was not going to be ruined by poop, yet I had to devise a plan to make a very quick getaway to the bathroom facilities as soon as the newly married couple exited the tent, all to be accomplished while attracting as little attention as possible. Oh the suspense of it all!

It must be understood that the ceremony was held in a beautiful outdoor setting. There was a wooden bridge that connected the mainland to a hillock where a white tent was set up for the ceremony and guests. The post-ceremony reveling tent and indoor reception facility that housed the washrooms were situated on the mainland. The ceremony ended, the bride, groom and their attendants had exited the tent, and were followed by the guests. This meant there was quite a lot of territory to cover, territory that was now filled with guests and I was a woman on the move. As it was my first time seeing many family members since the surgery, so many of whom had sent special cards, caring e-mails, loving phone calls, and fully cooked meals, they were lined up and ready to share with me their wonderful selves at this most auspicious occasion. I loved them all, wanted so much to thank each and every one of them, but I needed to get to that washroom. Quick! With Mark pushing me in the wheelchair as fast as the chair could move, together we felt as though we were running the gauntlet. As we speeded past the throng, we called out our hellos, gave our best smiles, occasional waves, and continued down the path. Over the bridge we went, scrambling down the walk to arrive at the washrooms. Blessed relief — or so I thought. Little did I know the fun was just beginning.

In what I believe to be the smallest cubical I have ever entered, I looked around to lay out my ostomy equipment. But the cubical had no flat surfaces, so I decided I could just simply place the purse on the floor, pull it wide open, and place the various pieces of equipment on it. *Aha, problem solved!* This being my first time dealing with my ostomy far away from the safety and my well-organized bathroom at home, I was unsure of how I was going to manage. Being the troopers Percy & Me are, we forged ahead.

Now it was time to hike up my pretty little top, and yank down my pants. Looking down at my abdomen, sure enough, I see the adhesive holding the flange was indeed peeling away from my skin. There was only the small barrier adhesive of the flange left holding the bag in place.

Oh, my. What am I going to do now? Oh, yes. I have a special belt in my kit that I can attach to each side of the flange, and which will help keep it in place. I congratulated myself for my resourceful thinking. As I had never attached it before, I was going to have to figure it out pretty quick. My top still hiked up, pants down around my ankles, ostomy supplies tucked under my arm, I rummage through my purse looking for my eyeglasses. I can't see close details without them. Can't find them in my @*# purse! Oh, wait. I have left them at home, I realized. This is okay, I can handle this. *Gosh, it's getting warmer in this non-air conditioned good-for-nothing micro-cubicle,* I grumbled to myself.

Placing the ostomy paraphernalia back on my purse, I unzipped the equipment pouch and reached in, taking out the special security belt. On both sides and at the top of the flange that is barely attached to my body by this time, are loops that the belt can be connected to. Unfortunately, everything is blurry (no glasses), and as I have never attached it before, I'm not sure how it actually attaches, but ready or not, here we go. Using my fingertips to feel things out, I began to attempt attaching the belt on the left side of the flange. *Gee, it's hot in this cubicle! Ah, there we go. Left side connected, now I'll just feed it around my waist and attach it to the right side . . .*

It was at this point I realized that because I had not put the belt on before, I had never sized it properly for my proportions. With another grumble, I removed the belt from the left side loop. I explored the belt with my fingers and was able to expand it. Time and time again I did this until it was the right size. All right, we're cooking with fire now.

With this, I began to once again feel the left side of the flange to locate the loop to hook the belt on. With it attached I fed the belt around the back of me and started to feel for the right side of the flange to locate the loop. It was at this time I suddenly remembered that we had been snipping off the right side flange loop up to this point to avoid injuring my still-healing surgery wound that runs from just above my belly button and six inches all the way down from there. *Oh, for @*# sake, what am I going to do now! Okay Jo-Ann, relax for a minute and think.* These words I repeated in my mind as I tried to calm myself.

Aha! I suddenly remembered, there is a loop at the top of the flange. I'll just attach the belt there. Once again, using my fingers to locate the loop and with perspiration dripping down my face, I found it. I was then able to attach the belt. Yahoo!

Unfortunately, the belt was now attached in such a way as to be on the left side of the flange and on the top of the flange rather than on the opposite right side. *Great! Now I look like some strange pirate who, instead of having a black patch over one eye, has a beige belly poop bag patch.* It was awkward and uncomfortable but as far as I could see, workable.

I started to arrange my outer clothing when all of a sudden there was a SPROING and the belt let go from the loop at the top of the flange, and then, within a split second, let go of the left hand loop and off it flew to the back corner behind the toilet with lightning speed.

Oh great! It was at this point that Mr Bean and the scene of him trying to change into his bathing suit on an open beach came to mind. (Mr. Bean is a British comedy written by and starring Rowan Atkinson as the title character. Mr. Bean is described as "a child in a grown man's body." Through physical humour, Mr Bean solves seemingly impossible problems presented by everyday tasks and often causes disruption in the process.)

As my mind filled with Mr. Bean's beach antics, it became difficult to suppress my giggles. Gathering my strength, which by this point was very quickly waning, and as I was slowly melting from the heat, I maneuvered down to my knees — quite a feat for me at that point in my healing journey. I leaned in, and somehow was able to reach and retrieve the ostomy belt.

With belt in hand, and feeling I'd accomplished a victory of sorts, I straightened up and was ready to start attaching my belt once again to the left hand and top loops on my flange. It was at this time, there came a knock on my micro-cubicle door, and a voice asked, "Are you OK? Can I help you with anything?"

"Oops. Uh. No thank you. I'm fine. But thank you," I answered sheepishly.

"You sure?" asked the lovely voice.

"No, I mean, yes. Thank you."

With as much determination and strength as I had left, I started feeling the left-hand side of the flange and attached the belt to it. I then attached the other end to the top loop, having had a lot of practice by this time. I pulled up my pants, lowered my top, and arranged my equipment back into my purse. I was now ready to partay!

With a wash of my hands, I shuffled out of the bathroom with a big smile on my face. Out the door I came and crumpled down into my wheelchair, hot, exhausted, and most pleased with myself. Mark asked me if everything had gone well and I just waved my hand and said, "Time to join the party, honey. Tell you about it later."

Illness Teaches Us How to Die, It Also Teaches Us How to Live

As I continued to recuperate from my long-term illness and lifesaving surgery, I had many dreams. One in particular stayed with me. During this dream I splished, sploshed and splashed through a landscape of thick and colourful semi-liquid substances. At one point in the dream I looked to my right and there, shiny in the sunlight, was a set of knives. Now, the knives were not aggressive in nature. They were simply shiny tools beside me. When I awoke, I could not shake the dream from my mind. As I thought deeply on it, I decided that the details meant something to me. Possibly my subconscious was trying to relay some message or messages to me. Dreams provide us with information symbolically. I realized that my inner self was trying to tell me something or some things.

Within a few days of thinking about the recurring dream, I realized the colourful and somewhat mucky substance throughout the dreamscape was all about texture. Well, Percy is all about texture, and right out there in front of me. The knives were quite easy to decipher. Surgical knives had been used to save my life as all the while they altered my physiology. With the expert hands of a surgeon, they had carved me into a survivor. Armed with these understandings, I realized, as part of my recovery, I would now take up oil painting with palette knives.

I had been a watercolour artist for a number of years. I decided through the message of my dreams it was time to change the medium. I went straight out and purchased oil paints, canvasses and palette knives. As I had never used this medium, nor painted with knives, I knew it would be quite the adventure.

I pondered what my first painting would be, and it dawned on me: since Percy has inspired me — and they say when an individual starts any new venture, one should start with what they know — I decided on "Percy, A Self-Portrait". Yes, I painted Percy. What I found out was that I absolutely love the oil medium. I can manipulate knives very well, and most importantly, the whole experience was, and continues to be, cathartic. Healing can be both fun and productive.

Still in recovery, I am slowly but surely building up my activity level. My mind is as busy as it always was although my body has a way to go still to catch up. Therefore, being able to paint and accomplish, was and is wonderful. Splishing, sploshing and splashing through the thick rainbow of colours using knives, has been very valuable to me emotionally, therefore physically as well.

I continued to paint with oil and knives, and for my next project I decided on a theme of doors and windows. Let's face it, a door (so to speak) was closed, and a window in the form of Percy was opened. So I chose to paint four large symbolic pictures. Each of these pictures features masonry walls with doors and windows, masonry walls being symbolic of the abdominal wall, and windows and doors representing the various entrances and exits of our human internal universe. Following these creations, my next set of pictures was created with Percy's ostomy opening in mind. These three smaller pictures depicted scenes within a circular porthole surrounded by solid painted backgrounds.

For a number of months, my creative muse consistently presented me with an odd visual thought in many ways both sad and most definitely unusual. As I pondered the landscapes of my mind, I realized there had been many times throughout the physical, emotional, and intellectual suffering (not to mention the stress on my human spirit) that I had experienced, through the illness, being brought to the brink of death. I would think: I feel as though my tears are of blood, and if I did cry tears of blood, I would bleed to death. In retrospect, this is an interesting feeling, and having shared it with other folks, I have found that many can relate to the depth of this level of pain and despair. I decided to bring out the oil paints and proceeded to create the scene. I painted this image experientially, emotionally and visually, for myself. Rather than using knives, I decided to paint it with a sponge, the ones people use to put on their makeup. I simply felt that using a sponge would be symbolic of soaking up tearful liquid. I also felt that the use of a makeup sponge was a metaphor for applying a mask, a mask which I did put on so many times to spare the hurt and worry of my loved ones who had to watch me descend into illness. Upon completion of the picture, I have come to the understanding that we as human beings, physically, emotionally, and mentally endure so very much. Living is not for wimps. I am considering my next artistic theme being that of paths. Paths in the forest, paths through a garden, and so forth. This outpouring reminds me of the new path in life that I am required to venture and navigate through. Life goes on. Life finds a way.

It was during this time that I was also writing this book. Through both of these activities, I was re-designing myself and my life. I was diving head first into my journey. It is so easy when one is very ill to believe that the glass is half empty. I'm not made that way. I much prefer to perceive myself and life as being at the very least half full. This way of viewing life does not necessarily come naturally to most of us. It is something we are required to create for ourselves, and then work very hard to achieve. My life has changed and some of what I have done before will not necessarily work anymore as I step into my future. I choose to step forward with awareness and with the desire to live the highest and best life possible for me and those who share my life. Therefore, I am using my creative activities as my tools for internal negotiations to build a new relationship with my altered self and life. I am integrating all of my systems to ensure emotional paralysis does not occur.

This approach is not new to me. Many years ago, when I was in my twenties, I fell seriously ill. The illness was not related to Percy. I underwent surgery that would alter my body and carve me into a survivor. It was my first major healing journey and it took almost a year to recuperate. At one point during my recovery, I noticed that the only topic of conversation I was having with those wonderful folks who visited me, was all about me and my illness.

"How are you feeling today?" "Can you move your left arm yet?" And so on, and so on.

I found these conversations to be boring, negative, and I sure didn't want them to be all about me. My mind was shrinking as small as my world had shrunk. I found that although I was delighted to see my visitors, when they left, I felt unsatisfied. I'm sure they did as well. That was it! I was going to find a way out of the doldrums. I was not going to wallow in my own misery and drag everyone else into the swamp with me. I decided I had to focus my attention on something else and move on.

After careful thought, I decided that my adventure would be to learn everything possible about butterflies. The power that Butterfly brings is for the mind, and the ability to know the mind or to change it. It is the art of transformation. Like the butterfly, I was at the egg stage, the beginning of my new self, my new normal. This was the stage where all had not yet become reality. Somehow, down the line I would enter the larval stage and this would be the time where I would have definitely made my decisions about my future. The cocoon stage would follow and this would be the time of developing Project Self. The final stage would be the stage of transformation, the leaving of my chrysalis state, and into my birth, my new life.

This approach proved beneficial for me and my special people in more ways than one. Being the time before Internet, folks who came to visit me delighted in going to the library and borrowing books on butterflies for me. They felt they were part of my healing transformation process. And they were! It gave us interesting things to discuss, moving the focus away from me and my illness. It put a metaphorical slant on my healing journey that was healthy and positive for everyone. As we discussed the symbology of Butterfly, I could then apply it to my healing journey as a positive and wonderful adventure. This sure uplifted me and my special ones.

The most important lesson I learned from Butterfly is that we and all things of this Universe are involved in a never-ending cycle of transformation.

Here I am again, in another part of the cycle of life, and this time I have Percy to share my life and this world with. We're writing and painting so we can release emotional tension. We are writing and painting so we may share our journey with those who may be interested. We are writing and painting so we can transform and transcend the alterations in the most self-enlightening manner possible. It's taking time and it takes a lot of work, but heck, it beats lying down, drying to dust and blowing away in the wind.

A joyful life is when we listen to the desires of our heart and mind, and we never forget to have a chuckle or two, a day. — Jo-Ann L. Tremblay

Percy's Poop Faux Pas

Bathroom adventures are a very large part of an ostomate's life. Most of us have had a lot of experience with bathrooms well before our ostomies were created. This as a result of folks who had suffered with various bowel diseases such as colitis, Crohn's disease, diverticulitis — the list goes on. Most of us spend many an hour locating and using all forms of bathrooms in all sorts of facilities on a frequent and urgent basis.

It was Mark's 62nd birthday and festivities included once again going to Maxwell's Bistro and Club. Yes, they let Jo-Ann out to play, finally. It was the second time that I had ventured out to such a busy public place since surgery. I even danced to a few tunes. (I was nervous on the dance floor as I was not too steady on my feet yet, and feared someone would inadvertently bump into Percy.)

A wonderful time was had by all. Percy was another story though, and I'll tell you about his poop faux pas shortly. The evening was particularly sweet as Mark, being a wonderful performer, song writer, singer, and guitarist, and so, for his birthday, performed live with the band. It sure was nice dancing to the sweet sounds of Johnny Vegas, the band, Beki and my hubby.

Now as for Percy, well . . . We have to be a little patient with him. Let's face it, at that time he was only four months old. With all of the great food, dancing and so on,

Percy became quite excited and decided he would like to be active as well. So inevitably, Percy & Me had to head to the public washroom. Now don't get me wrong, Maxwell's is a very clean and well-appointed bistro/club, but it is public. I was a bit concerned as to how Percy & Me were going to do our business. Interestingly, all the material I have read describes how one would work things out on a clean toilet, but nothing I have read so far talks about a public one. "Gee, I don't want to sit on that kind of toilet." So Percy being very active, and I not wanting to touch any surfaces, we thought we had worked out a plan. As you know how best laid plans of men and mice can go, despite all our good planning, Percy & Me found ourselves out of step with one another and out of alignment with the toilet. Next thing we know, Percy has a projectile moment. I am caught by surprise so a lovely dollop of poop lands right on the top of my lovely beige suede left foot boot. Oops! After some suppressed giggles on my part, wind breaking on Percy's part, we work out our toilet detail. We then proceeded to the sink to rescue my suede boot all the time I'm thinking that I had really wanted to buy the chocolate brown ones, but oh no, I bought the neutral beige-goes-with-everything ones. The boots ended up looking pretty good, and I'd work with them further.

Happy Anniversary, Honey

Mark and I were married later in life. Mark has often joked, "Oh, honey, some day it may be that we'll have to wipe each other's bottoms." Little did we know it would come sooner than we thought.

Three thirty in the morning of our 5th wedding anniversary, I was startled from a deep sleep by a most uncomfortable feeling. As I slowly awakened, it became very apparent that I'd had an equipment malfunction. As you can imagine, the contents of the bag were all over me, my pajamas, and the sheets. I carefully lifted myself from the bed and made my way to the bathroom. As I turned on the light, I realized that some of the brown mess was now also on our powder-blue bedroom rug. Mark, now fully awake, looked around, most definitely sniffed, and his eyes met my eyes. *What a mess!* was my only thought.

While I was cleaning myself up, Mark looked at me with a gentle smile on his face as he removed the sheets from the bed, took my pajamas, and headed down to the basement to put them into the washing machine. On his way up the stairs, he stopped off in the kitchen and filled a bowl with cleaning soap for the rug and up the stairs he came.

When I had finished in the bathroom, I went into the bedroom and bent down to my hands and knees and started cleaning the rug, with tears streaking down my cheeks. Mark stood silently beside me, ready to help out in any way possible.

It was at this time I remembered it was our wedding anniversary. I looked up, gave Mark a feeble smile and said, "Happy Anniversary, honey."

In a gentle voice, he said, "Happy Anniversary, babe," then he turned around, got fresh clean sheets from the linen closet, and put them on the mattress. As he crawled into bed once again, he leaned over and with smile on his face gave me a kiss, curled up and went back to sleep.

Mommy-sitting

Through the aftermath of surgery and during the healing process, primary caregivers are amazing. They keep the home as organized as possible under the circumstances. They cater to their patients' physical, emotional, medical, and intellectual needs as they assist in keeping everyone's spirits up. They are our advocates between the doctors and nurses, they arrange appointments, and the list goes on. Day and night they are on duty with very little time for taking care of their own needs. And so, it is important that they get a break. They need to take time for themselves and simply just get away from it all from time to time. Mark is a true fan of live music and so it has been healthy for him to be able to get a break from his caregiving duties to enjoy himself and the music that fills him. This is where my son, Richard, stepped up to the plate. Richard leaves his little family to spend the evening with me.

My health issues during a large part of my recovery were many and it was unadvisable that I should be left alone. Richard and I spent the hours together watching interesting television shows, and at other times talked about anything and everything. Although one does not want to be in the situation I was in, nor want their child who works full time, is a husband and a father, to feel he must leave his home to "mommy-sit", those hours have been precious to me. I am fortunate to have had the opportunity to spend wonderful moments with the special people in my life. It makes me feel as though I have captured life itself.

Scaredy-cat

Having a colostomy situated in the abdomen beside a belly button is an amazing invention. It gives us a second chance at life. But let's be real, it is completely unnatural.

This reality came to light when one day I was standing in the doorway between one of the bedrooms and our TV room. My cat, Niki, was relaxing on the couch. She stretched luxuriously and looked over at me. It was at this time that Percy — not having any social graces — chose to pass wind. It was quite loud and sounded like a balloon that has not been tied off and is now letting go of air. Poor Niki. She sprang to her feet then crouched down low with her ears pinned back as she stared past me into the bedroom. With eyes open wide she awaited the loud terrible monster that she was sure was lurking there. As I doubled over laughing and giving her reassuring pets on her head, I was reminded of how I and my life had changed in so many ways.

Percy Goes to Florida

Traveling is one of my favourite things to do. I have been very fortunate to have travelled to just about everywhere on our planet with the exception of Antarctica. Being so ill for the past few years, I was unable to travel anywhere, and this was disconcerting. With the illness dragging on, then the emergency surgery and the creation of Percy, I had been unable to travel for what felt like a very long time. It was a wonderful day when my doctor gave me the all-clear to begin traveling. We were very excited indeed!

Doing anything with an ostomy is a challenge and one must do a lot of upfront planning. It certainly is not insurmountable, but it's a challenge no less. There are many sources of information that provide traveling with an ostomy tips and suggestions. There are forums where people with ostomies share their experiences via stories about traveling and offer advice for planning a trip. There are listings for ostomy contacts around the world. There is even a free service that will provide key words and phrases translated into more than eleven languages in the event an ostomate traveller might require support in the foreign country.

It was decided that our first travel adventure needed to be very civilized with all the conveniences of home. I was still in recovery mode. It was January and since we live in cold snowy Ottawa, we were sunny-Florida-bound. Our destination was a lovely condominium in Naples, Florida, which we would share with our sister, brother-in-law, and their daughter, Lia.

Preparing for our vacation started a month before air flight departure from Ottawa to Fort Myers.

During this time, I continued to explore the ostomates' travel forums for good tips, suggestions, and important information. All suggested locating the closest United Ostomy Association branch in the area we would be staying at, making sure to have the contact names and the emergency volunteer phone number; also to ensure we had the address and contact information of the closest medical/ ostomy supplier. We did this. Suggestions also included ensuring that the ostomate bring double the equipment supplies that would be required for the duration of the stay.

Percy the Bag Bomber

It was now time to research Flying With Percy. A young ostomate in the United States placed a very informative YouTube video sharing her flying experience with a focus on security screening. Her suggestion was to bring your supplies with you in your carry-on luggage in the event that somehow your luggage got lost. You would have all of your required supplies with you. She also relayed that when flying at a couple of airports, in her experience, she was required to undergo a more-extensive security search. This meant she had to run her fingers around the waistband of her underwear, after which a security representative wiped her hands with a special tissue and this was placed into a scanning machine to detect if there were any bomb residue. The security officer then will do the same thing. With this completed, she was then off to enjoy her flight. The young lady also recommended that the ostomate go onto the Transportation Security Administration (TSA) website. On that site, there is a Notification Card one can download, fill out with the appropriate information and which then can be laminated. I put one card in my wallet and my husband put a duplicate card in his wallet. This card basically states: TSA respects the privacy concerns of all members of the traveling public. This card allows you to describe your health condition, disability or medical device to the TSA officer in a discrete manner. Presenting the card does not exempt you from screening. The travel card is helpful to identify your supplies at Customs inspections.

As my research continued to reveal information, it came to light that sometimes our ostomy bags can inflate to a certain extent due to the pressure change in the plane. Well, this set off some comical scenes in my head. I imagined myself reaching a 35,000-foot cruising altitude when all of a sudden Percy's bag would become so inflated the seams would burst, and I was now zooming throughout the plane's cabin like a deflating balloon and with fecal matter being flung around splatting onto my innocent and unsuspecting fellow travelers. *What a sight!*

Not wanting to be a bag bomber, I continued my research. It was suggested that the ostomate not drink fizzy liquids twenty-four to forty-eight hours prior to flying. It was also suggested not to eat gas-producing foods prior to or during the flight.

I was anxious, this was to be my first vacation away from home as an ostomate. I was so inexperienced and now had the added fear of being a bag bomber but Percy, Mark, and I embarked on our Florida adventure.

When I entered airport security, I provided my notification card, each of the security representatives thanked me for informing them. They stated that as long as I did not set off any of the metal detector equipment, they would not request further security inspection. I very much appreciated their discretion and even for expressing their gratitude to me for bringing Percy and the ostomy equipment to their attention.

The big moment for me came when the plane left the runway and we began to climb to higher and higher altitudes. With bag bomber images running through my head, I waited nervously until we reached our cruising altitude. Percy's bag did not inflate, did not blow off the flange, and I am glad to say it was a smooth and uneventful flight to Florida.

Say What?

Over time and with experience, an ostomate will know that sometimes — even with the best of equipment and attention to our ostomy — there will be accidents. Understandably, these can be very disconcerting so we do our best, of course, to avoid them.

Here we were on vacation, all nestled in our comfy condominium. I had purchased a special light-blue incontinence bed-pad to be placed under the bed-sheet to protect the mattress in the event I had an ostomy equipment failure. Ah, my trendy and fashionable ostomate accessories!

Being on vacation away from home, my usual foods, local water and my daily routine, I must say I was anxious as to how my body and Percy would react. Over the days, I did have some physical issues and had to deal with them. As a result, I was very pleased that I had brought along the additional mattress protector. The worst that would happen is that I would have to wash the sheets.

But, as you can imagine, I was not as confident in the bed during the night as I usually had been before Percy was born. We were having a wonderful vacation, my strength and stamina were building. The fresh fruit, vegetables, vitamin D from the sun, relaxation and so on, were just what the doctor ordered. By the third night, I had finally fully relaxed and fell into a deep and wonderful slumber.

When all of a sudden I could hear my husband's voice saying something to me in a forceful manner. As I shook the grogginess from my head, I distinctly heard Mark say, "You stink."

"What?"

"You're stinking, Jo-Ann."

Oh, no. My nightmare had materialized. I must have had an equipment failure and the bed was a mess. Panic set in and I rose up from the bed, cupped my ostomy bag in both my hands and ran to the bathroom saying, "Oh no, oh no!" Upon arrival in the bathroom I inspected myself, Percy, and the equipment, but could not find any reason why I would be stinky. After a while of checking and re-checking, I returned to the bedroom and said to Mark, "I don't understand why I stink. I've checked everything and nothing's wrong."

That's when he said, "I didn't say you're stinking, I said you're snoring."

Let 'Er Rip

Driving from Ottawa to just east of Toronto to visit our newest granddaughter takes about four hours. There are the obligatory full-service rest stops including fuel, washrooms, food services, and convenience stores along the 401 highway.

As it was around lunch time, we decided to grab a snack at one of the not-so-good, but oh-so-quick fast food counters. We ate a satisfactory lunch, stopped one more time to empty our bladders, and on the road we went once again.

About twenty minutes later, my intestines, or at least what's left of them, began to gurgle and bubble and I began to feel somewhat uncomfortable. The gurgles gurgled even louder and with more frequency. I undid the button of the waistband of my slacks.

And with the pressure of an oil rig, my ostomy bag began to fill. In ten seconds flat, the ol' bag was about to blow!

"Oh, no! Mark! I need a toilet. NOW!"

Well we were in the middle of nowhere yet we had to be close to somewhere. A sign indicated we could exit the main highway and enter a little town. Percy's bag was full to capacity, and I knew we were at the, let-'er-rip point. Down the exit ramp we travelled. We reached a T intersection, the town to our left and a few more kilometres down the secondary road.

"Oh gosh, I'm going to have a real mess soon, Mark. Poop is going to hit the fan!" Panic was setting in and beads of sweat dripped down my face. Anxiety filled, I began to have visions dancing in my head of brown splat all over the front of me.

Geez. Does this town even exist? How far do we have to go? My mind raced helter skelter. By now, my slacks were completely unbuttoned, the zipper completely opened, and Percy's bag at fuller than full capacity. Not a pretty sight.

Finally, a privately owned fuel station and little convenience store appeared around the bend. "MARK! Here's a place. Stop here. NOW!" Poor Mark. Maneuvering the car around the bend in the road at a quick pace, he was able to pull off the road and up to the little station.

Bunching the front and top of my slacks with my left hand to make sure they did not fall to my ankles, I grabbed my sweater with my right hand and pulled it down low to cover my exposed abdomen and Percy, and I ran as best I could into the little bathroom. Not the picture of elegance you can be sure.

Relief for that very brief moment had only started to settle my nerves. As I sidled up to the toilet, I realized that I had to step back again and do a reconnoitre. The room was extremely small. Here we go again with the undersized facilities. Just my luck! I did not have much time left, Percy's bag needed immediate attention, but there was something different about this facility. I realized that the room had been built on two levels. The lower level was the entrance to the room. The sink to my right was on the lower level. The toilet itself was perched up on a second level about four inches higher. Unfortunately, the front of the toilet was placed about two inches away from the edge of the step. This meant I could not stand at the front of the toilet to deal with Percy's bag on the same level as the toilet.

Where there's a will, there's a way. There is a solution to everything. Think Jo-Ann, think. So, I tried to move to the side of the toilet, but the walls were so close, no one, not even a child, could fit between the wall and the toilet on that level. As I am only 4'11", there was no way to stand at the front of the toilet on the lower level and aim to attend to Percy. I am simply too short.

Meanwhile I must give praise to Percy's equipment, it still held, a miracle perhaps. Grabbing hand drying paper from the dispensary as quickly as possible I placed some on the floor, and then did my best to empty as much of the contents of the ostomy bag as possible into the toilet as I could. Visions of the sometimes irate monkeys at the zoo hurling stuff certainly came to mind, if you know what I mean.

About ten minutes later, I emerged from the small fuel station and to the car where Mark was patiently waiting for me. Wet with sweat still, but with buttoned-up slacks, I stumbled into the car, and with a frown on my face I said, "What a bizarre bathroom. I think Percy & Me have seen it all now. I'll have to do a little washing load when we get to the kids'."

This experience has helped me realize how resourceful one can be in the strangest of circumstances, and as they say, "don't sweat the small stuff". I would also like to say, if you are planning to install a toilet on a higher level than the main floor, please ensure you give enough room for an adult to stand either in front of it, or beside it. Thank you.

PART 4

Fragile, Limited, Precious

One year ago today I underwent life-saving surgery. Today is my Celebration of Life Day. It's my second chance, the bonus, the icing on the cake, the cherry on top. My first chance was amazing, my second chance incredible. Life is fragile, limited and precious. Always have had the time of my life, why not, it's the only life I thought I had. Now, with a second chance, I am having the time of my life, why not, it's the only life I know *I have. Thank you everyone who has travelled the illness and healing journey with me. Thank you, Mark, for everything and all the beyonds you've been and done for me. Thank you, Richard, for all that you are.* — Forever-grateful Jo-Ann

You are part of the fabric of your personal and professional community, country, and world. When you actualize your potentials in your own unique way, our world actualizes its potential, too. — Jo-Ann L. Tremblay

Poopology

The art of pooping is a subject many people would rather not discuss. Most of us don't want to admit that we poop. Many feel it's all too-much-information. The fact remains that pooping is imperative to our health, life can not exist without it. What enters our body is important, how it is processed, then what's left over, and that which exits our bodies, is very important.

It's time to put the poop on poops out there and on everyone's mind. Colon cancer is reported to be 90% circumventable if detected early. In 2011, an estimated 22,200 new cases were diagnosed in Canada. Close to 8,900 Canadians lost their lives that same year. Estimated new cases in the United States in 2011 were 103,170 colon cancer and 40,290 rectal cancer. Deaths in that year were 51,690 colon and rectal cancer combined. Our pooper equipment needs regular checkups no matter how uncomfortable we may feel about this.

Have fun, study the how, the where and the what about poop. Find out where poop comes from. Explore how poop is made. Hey, be an environmentalist and find out where poop goes after you flush, if that's your fancy. Whatever your interest, what's important is to bring poop out of the dark recesses of the outhouse. No more tunnel vision (pardon the pun), and widen your perspective and knowledge about poop. Bring poop out into the light of day. You might save your own life or someone else's some day, and that is a fact.

Children don't have as much of a problem with poop, so let's educate them from the very beginning. A number of years ago, when my son was about eight years old, my sister and I took him and his two cousins to a poop exhibition at the Royal Ontario Museum in Toronto. The kids went wild. They loved it. With giggles, yelps and break-down belly laughs, they examined the difference between the feces of our ancient relatives and the feces of our own North American modern-day population. The example feces of our ancient relatives had texture and the make up of it was quite thick, grainy and pasty. This was a result of eating natural foods filled with bulk, grains, fibre, and goodness knows whatever else our ancient relatives could find to eat. Our modern day feces on the other hand have a smooth texture resembling tooth paste. Hmm. Quite a difference, and a result of eating our highly processed foods. The children, who are now all grown up and have children of their own, still remember the poop exhibition. They were not em-bare-assed, they saw the humour, and learned a great deal about the digestive system and how it works. They learned about food. Basically what goes in, how it's processed, and what comes out — and so did I. The poop on poops is important. It can affect one's long-term health, and can't be mentioned enough times. So raise a glass of your favourite wine whose grapes were probably fertilized by some form of poop, or clink a mug of your favourite brew whose hops were probably fertilized by some other form of poop, and celebrate the value of caring, paying attention to, and sharing the poop on poops.

Ostomates

In Part 2 of this book, I briefly talked about "Cool Dudes & Dudettes", and I would like to expand on these wonderful folks and what they do. I'm referring to the members of the United Ostomy Association of Canada Inc. (UOAC). The UOAC is a volunteer-based organization dedicated to assisting all persons facing life with gastrointestinal or urinary diversions by providing emotional support, experienced and practical help, instructional and informational services throughout its membership and to the family unit, associated caregivers, and the general public.

Support is not only available to Canadians, there is the International Ostomy Association (IOA). It has been created as an organization of ostomy associations dedicated to improving the life of ostomates around the globe. Worldwide associations include the Asia South Pacific Ostomy Association (ASPOA) which has regional ostomy associations for both Asia and the South Pacific countries, and which advocates quality of life for all ostomates. There is the European Ostomy Association (EOA) and the Ostomy Association of the Americas (OAA) who complement and strengthen each other by promoting the rights of ostomates, quality patient care, and also by providing support and medical know-how for ostomates and health professionals world wide.

Each of these associations has a quest to promote ostomy advocacy for people who have undergone life-saving and life-changing surgery to live a normal life in society. These organizations bring to the attention of the general public the needs and aspirations of ostomates. They provide support, important information, and address the needs of and offer support to ostomates, significant others, their caregivers, advocates, and family and friends. This is done through different activities such as educational programs, seminars and support meetings. They promote themselves through the use of mass media like newspaper and magazine announcements, advertisements and articles. The publication of informative handout materials and brochures, personal visits and lobbying activities are important tools toward helping promote the advocacy. Others seek official government proclamations and joint activities with allied agencies and professional health associations to further the cause.

Volunteers provide information and support for spouses and significant others. There are information pamphlets. There are partner support program through which spouses and significant others of new ostomates are made aware that help and support is available for them, as well. Volunteers man the phones for any emergency calls that may come. Spouses and significant others of ostomates and ostomates themselves can decide to take courses and become trained visitors who are then prepared to offer help and support to those who request it. Each association meets to discuss and share concerns, ideas and solutions.

There are young adult groups designed to offer a forum to those persons with ostomies who would like to meet with others in a similar age group to share ideas, develop friendships and learn more about living with an ostomy. It is open to all young adults, regardless of type of ostomy or alternate procedure, sexual orientation or marital status. Young ostomates can get together and swap stories, trade ostomy secrets and learn more about being a young adult with an ostomy.

There is the Parents of Children with Ostomy group. Yes, there are babies who have ostomies. There are children of all ages who are ostomates. From youth camp experiences, friendships, to advocacy, children and their families are offered support.

As you read, you are gaining the understanding that bowel disease has no boundaries. It does not care what gender you are, how old you are, what your ethnicity is. Everyone is vulnerable. And everyone has an equal opportunity to suffer from bowel disease and its attendant complications.

I would also like to mention at this time, no matter what your situation in life, whether you have a bowel disease, a heart condition, Hep C, if you're a hemophiliac, or you are a caregiver or advocate for someone in need, there are associations in your region dedicated to support and advocacy. You are not alone. You are not an island. You are not adrift. You are surrounded by people who are just like you, people who understand what you have gone through, and what you are going through now. Seek them out, give them a try. You deserve all the support, up-to-date information, and full access to whatever you require today and in the future.

Cottage Bound: 31 Mile Lake, Quebec Canada

It's just about July 1, 2012 and we're on our way to the cottage. Looking back at the past year I can only think, wow, the last time we were at the cottage was a year ago, almost to the day. It was a year ago my illness was moving along at a fast pace and I was very ill. I had been spending most of my days and evenings in a supine position. I had lost a lot of weight, and had no strength or body fat left. I was exhausted. On that July 1 in 2011, Mark and I were invited to our sister and brother-in-law's cottage. I am an outdoor person, and being in the wilderness and sharing time with our beloved family was so tempting, that although I was so ill, it was off to the cottage by the lake for us. I had figured if I were going to die, I couldn't think of a better place to do it, nor better people to be the last folks I saw on this Earth. We had loved our four days at the cottage. I had spent a lot of time in the outhouse with a beautiful view of the lake. I had developed a severe limp. But I'd had a wonderful time.

This day, as we entered the boreal forest along the dirt road, memories of the year before flooded back. Once again, we were spending time with our beloved family in the wilderness surrounded by nature and by the lake. Heaven on Earth. I realized that some of my excitement was because I had actually survived. I had been only an hour from death. I had the emergency surgery that prompted the physician to urge Mark and I to say our goodbyes. My amputation has created Percy, for better or for worse. The truth of the matter is, Percy & Me have been given a chance to venture out into paradise. We live on a beautiful planet.

Earth is amazing. And along with my pal, Percy, for as long as it lasts, we're on an adventure together.

A Promise

I promised myself that I would write my recovery story until Percy's 1st anniversary date. Today is July 21, 2012. My goodness, a year already. Time can go so fast. In the weeks leading up to my Celebration of Life Day, I have been preparing. I wanted to have a special celebration, and I wasn't sure what it would be. After some thought, I decided to paint oil miniatures that I would give to people who would be with me on the special day. On the back of each little canvas I wrote the following dedication: "This oil painting has been created and given to you with love in celebration of life, from Percy, Mark and me." Each of the twelve paintings was a labour of love, and depicted various scenes of life, from landscapes, the ocean and sunsets, to stormy skies. They are vignettes of the many life-wonders we see, smell, hear, taste, and touch every day.

With these completed, I then decided that Percy would be dressed in his party best. I went to the store and purchased self-stick gems. I created a fireworks burst design and applied them to Percy's poop bag. He sparkled with bling.

I baked confetti cupcakes, iced them in white and sprinkled them with coloured candy. Each would have a little birthday candle to be lit for a wish to be granted. My grandson, Evan, thought this was a great idea.

We then received a call from our friend Johnny Vegas, reminding us that he and pianist Eddie Bimm would be performing at Mooney's Bay Bistro on July 21. Wow. Isn't life amazing? My journey with Percy started with Johnny Vegas and his All Star Band performing at Maxwell's Bistro and Club, July 21, 2011, and my first year was ending with Johnny Vegas and Eddie performing. What were the odds? Was it destined? Was it fated to play out this way? I'll never know the answer, but I was certainly delighted to celebrate our special day with Johnny, Eddie, Mark, and the rest of the folks who dined with us while they listened to wonderful music.

I gave away the paintings to everyone around me. I ate scrumptious food. I delighted in the music. And Percy & Me are at peace with each other and our world.

When in Doubt, Just Take the Next Small Step

We all have a long road ahead of us. I know life isn't fair, but it's still good, and when I'm in doubt — which happens from time to time — I have learned to just take the next small step. I've heard folks who want to help others cope with life say, "Frame every so-called disaster with these words — in five years, will this matter?" Well, my response is, "YES," it all matters. My descent to the brink of death followed by my ascent to my new normal — and everything in between — matters.

How long our lives will be, no one really knows. Every one of us lives a life that is not always peaceful. The journey of life will not always be smooth. We cannot control life but we sure can control ourselves within every one of our life expressions and experiences. The things of life that we cannot control, we can certainly use as inspiration. In this way, we can make those life experiences that are good and not so good an ongoing process of discovery. If we have to go through it anyway, and certainly some of it is pretty awful, why not create something valuable out of it all? In this way, we don't feel so hard-done-by, we don't feel so much the victim. Instead, we can touch something precious within ourselves, be our own hero if need be.

Many folks have experienced illness, debilitating situations, or have come near to experiencing death. In my case, at this time in my life, it was due to my bowels. We all have a story to tell. We go through shock, denial, suffering, anger, profound sadness, and gratitude that we are alive. Sometimes we feel this kaleidoscope of emotions as we simultaneously begin to reconstruct our lives. Some of us start finding food to be more tasty. For some, the air they have been given a second chance to breath becomes fresher. There's a host of other things that being human and living life brings. No one is perfect, nevertheless, if we stay in the process of learning, growing and developing, this will become the common thread that binds all thoughts, behaviours, and actions. It is within this tapestry that we can see who we are, what we are doing, and where we eventually want to go in life, one step at a time. This is our life healing process.

My grandmother lived to be over 100 years old. Toward the end of her time with us on Earth, although her mind was still as sharp as a tack, her body was beginning to fail her. We had many long conversations during these years. It must have been a particularly bad day for me, as I complained to her. It was something along the lines of feeling I was working too hard, and I was obviously feeling sorry for myself. In her loving and gentle way she chastised me, and put some good common sense back into my head. She started by saying "I was born in 1895. I worked hard all my life, harder than you can imagine, and I'm still here. Hard work will not kill you, Jo-Ann. In fact, it is really important that you understand that hard work is good for you. Although I am unable to do what I did before, I'm still not finished working. From my wheelchair and sometimes from my bed, I work hard at praying for the very ill and infirm. This is my work now. This is what I can do at my age. So, Jo-Ann, I had days that there just wasn't enough hours, there were the times when I was very ill and I wasn't sure what lay ahead of me, it was in those times of doubt that I just took one small step at a time. That has always worked for me. I think you might want to give it a try."

Well, my grandmother had many wisdoms she shared, but this wisdom has come to mind for me over this past year during my healing journey many times. As with any illness, our job is to recover. As with any surgery, our job is to heal. As with any disability, our job is to be resourceful. As with our caregivers during these times when we feel weak and vulnerable, our job is to surrender to their integrity, desire and actions as our advocates. All the while, even when we are in doubt, we can just take one small step at a time. With each step we continue our journey of life.

Better with a Bag than in a Bag

After a year living with Percy, I no longer feel physically terrible. I have regained control of my life. Although I continue to live with the ravages left from the original disease, some complications from the extensive surgery, the ongoing everyday physical realities of living without a part of my large bowel, and with Percy, through it all, I have regained control of my life. A life that is forever changed.

Sitting here at my computer now, a whole year has passed and I feel I am living another life, in another world. I have taken the thoughts, feelings and experiences of the past year and put them onto paper. I had hoped this would help me have a better understanding of what happened to me. My desire was to allow it all to pour out of my mind and body so that I would not have to carry the weight of it around for the rest of my days. I dared to wish that I would be able to make sense of it as I stepped out into my new life, my new normal.

Truth be told, trying to make sense of it no longer bothers me as much has it had at first. Well . . . It still feels all rather senseless to me, but I guess it is what it is. What I do know: certain things happen because of bad genes, bad luck, wrong diagnoses, misplaced trusts, and as matter of fact, in *all* lives, shit happens. Bad things happen to bad people and bad things happen to good people. That's life.

During this past year, countless folk have continued to state "It all happens for a reason." "There's more for you to do." "You're not meant to go yet." That's what they say. Still makes me laugh, makes me cry, makes me angry, and mostly it makes me think. There still are times when all I want to do is to forget all of this happened. I want to wake up from the bad dream. There are times when I still get jaw-dropping amazed and my mind is blown when I think of what has transpired over the past five years. In the final analysis, I am responsible and accountable for making a reason out of what I have gone through. I am responsible and accountable for doing something(s) good and positive as a result of it all. And yes, obviously, I'm alive. I have consciously and purposely shone a light on my journey before Percy's creation and during our recovery, and shared the poop on poops. Percy & Me certainly hope you've had a chuckle or two on us, and that we have inspired you to celebrate who you are. Thank you for joining us on the path of life. No matter what happens as we journey forward, we know from now on, it's in the bag.

Epilogue

My life is saved and Percy has joined me on this odyssey.

It's July 22, 2012, the day after the first anniversary of my lifesaving surgery, and my Celebration of Life Day is now history. The candles have been blown out, the cupcakes devoured, Percy's gem-studded bag has been thrown away. Time to move on — or so I thought. As I look forward to my future, on the horizon there's another storm brewing.

"Oh, another surgery, you say." I repeated the doctor's statement as a queasy feeling slowly spread through my stomach and down my legs.

"Yes, the Modified Sugarbaker Technique," she said.

Wow, they sure come up with some doozy names. Must be their way of sugar-coating so their patients don't faint from fear.

"We will open your abdomen again from your belly button down, then we'll head in for the repair . . ." The doctor's voice started fading, as my brain got fuzzy. "We'll insert a mesh. Percy will be in a type of sling . . ."

Where does this real-life story go?

The adventures continue! ***Better WITH a Bag than IN a Bag: The Sequel*** is scheduled to be released in 2014.

Acknowledgments

Where do I begin, where do I end? There are so many folks to acknowledge and to thank. We are on an healing adventure of a lifetime, Percy & Me have never been alone, you are all with us on this journey. Thank you.

We would like to start by expressing our gratitude at the very beginning, and then step forward along our path of recovery.

Mark Henderson, my life partner for your belief in me, and your amazing support. Thank you for you.

Richard Tremblay, my son, you are my rock.

Dr Chinedu Onochie, Internal Medicine, for your professional expertise, relentless pursuit for definitive diagnosis, pulling together healing teams, and for consistent and compassionate follow-up.

Rebecca Auer, MD, Msc, FRCSC, Surgical Oncologist at the Ottawa Hospital-General Campus, for heading the operating theatre team, and successfully carving me into a survivor.

Ottawa Hospital-General Campus, thank you reception staff for prompt and expert frontline care.

Ottawa Hospital-General Campus Emergency Department – in gratitude for the Doctors and Nurses, you are a synchronized action team. All of you stabilized vitals, instilled trust and confidence during the frightening and uncertain hours leading to life saving surgery.

Rebecca Lantos, in appreciation for your administrative expertise in assisting Mark in navigating the bureaucracy.

Ottawa Hospital-General Campus floor nurses team and support staff. Thank you for your gentle administrations. I always felt I was in capable healing hands throughout my hospital stay.

The Ontario Home Care Nurses. You were resourceful professionals with that personal touch. Thank you for your calmness and ingenuity in getting us through administrative snafus. You calmed our nerves and helped us know we had strong advocates committed to getting us on the road to recovery.

Ostomy Equipment Suppliers, hotline support. I am grateful for your assistance in helping me find the ostomy appliances that work for me. And, for guiding me through the myriad of options available. You are all highly professional and caring.

Shawna Croteau, Senior Home Healthcare Sales Consultant, Ontario Medical Supply, for your expertise in assisting Percy, Me and Mark, navigate the sometimes confusing world of colostomy equipment. Your patience and winning smile, is greatly appreciated.

Crowe Creations, Sherrill Wark, Editor. Thank you for ensuring this book made its way to publication with all the t's crossed, and i's dotted. Your support is so greatly appreciated.

Andre (Andy) Manson, ET Nurse/Ostomy Care and Supply Centre, New Westminster, Canada - thank you for your hernia belt expertise, and ensuring Percy and Me had the right fit. Also, thank you for all the support.

Carol Stephen, award winning poet and fellow ostomate, my venting partner and friend, thank you for all your support, and putting up with my, "oh I'm so grumpy today", e-mails.

Mike MacDonald, one of Canada's Premier Comedians – laughter is a great medicine, it is the healer and the cosmic glue that binds us all. Thank you and God Bless.

Last and not least: I beg forgiveness of all those who have been with me over the course of the years and whose names I have failed to mention.

About the Author

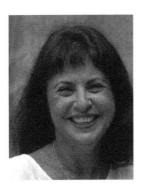

Jo-Ann L. Tremblay, is a personal/professional life coach, trainer, photographer, and water colour/oil artist. She is the author of **The Self-Coaching Toolbox – Six tools for personal and professional growth & development.** Jo-Ann has created and hosted the television special, *That's Life*, hosted 2 television program series – and a radio program series, *Voices of Our Town*.

After a lengthy illness Jo-Ann underwent life saving surgery that resulted in the creation of a descending colostomy, she affectionately calls, "Percy".

Now an ostomate, Jo-Ann L. Tremblay, joins in with fellow ostomates, their caregivers, medical experts and people in general, with a mix of humour, inspiration, and a large dollop of empathy, in celebration of second chances at creating and living a joyous quality of life, in spite of it all.

Website: www.potentialsmanagement.com
Blog: joannltremblay.wordpress.com
Twitter: @joanntremblay

Other Books by Jo-Ann L. Tremblay

The Self-Coaching Toolbox

ISBN 1-897113-06-4

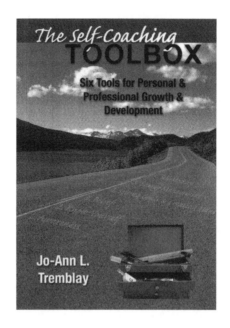

Available for purchase at

General Store Publishing House

www.gsph.com

Printed in Great Britain
by Amazon